STETHOSCOPE STORIES

A FANCIFUL MEMOIR OF THE LIFE AND TIMES OF A COUNTRY DOCTOR

BY

JOE COPPOLA, M.D.

STETHOSCOPE STORIES

A FANCIFUL MEMOIR OF THE LIFE AND TIMES OF A COUNTRY DOCTOR

A McKinney Publishing Production
Printing History: First Edition, December 2019

Cover Photo: *School-itis.* by Norman Rockwell. Originally published on the cover of *Leslie's* magazine, October 5, 1916.

ISBN: 978-1-943518-29-6

For information address:

McKinney Publishing
4261 E. University Dr. #30-312
Prosper, TX 75078

Visit our website at:
WWW.McKinneyPublishing.com

McKinney PUBLISHING

This book is dedicated to my faithful and loving wife,
without whom I could not have endured,
and to my children, who taught me what it means to be a
father and whom I would sometimes embarrass.

INTRODUCTION

This book is a work of fiction based on actual events. The format is whimsical and in vignette style. The stories are not necessarily chronological nor in any meaningful order. Almost all the names and places have been changed to protect both the innocent and the guilty. Some characters may be a fusion of two or more people, and the conversations related may or may not have actually happened with the persons mentioned. But most of them happened as described. Observations, conclusions and assumed or shared thoughts are strictly my own, and may bear no resemblance to reality. The purpose of this book is primarily for entertainment, and to give a small degree of insight into a profession that is more art than science, to show how medicine was practiced in a time that has past and to show what living in a small town was like. I hope you read this as it was written, looking for the humorous, the poignant, the lasting and the soul searching.

Preface

In the summer of 1976 I had finished my residency in Family Medicine and was ready to start my own practice. A professional life, whether in medicine, law, teaching or what have you, is much like seasons. It starts in the spring, with great expectations. Ideals are planted and some bloom like the flowers of spring, while some die. You plant, fertilize, water and nurture your newly formed profession. You put in long hours. You weed out what is choking it, and feed that which is growing it. As you watch it grow, you think all growth is good, but it is only later that you find that all growth is not a blessing. The blessings come, not from growth, but from the individual relationships that are forged.

Then comes summer, when it warms up. The days are long, and the practice begins to run you, rather than you running it. You have a hard time keeping up with it, and one day blends into another. Time passes at a blinding speed. Weeks turn into months and months into years, and you don't know how the time has gotten away from you. You would hardly remember what year it was if you didn't have to write the date every day. It is always just one more patient to see, one more call to make, one more admission to do. Whatever gains you achieve in your practice activity, you lose in time and relationships. You don't realize the high price you pay for your time. You think you have more time than money. What you don't realize is that you can earn more money, but time, once gone, is gone forever. However at the time you don't realize the cost of a "successful" practice is an unfulfilled family life. It is only later that you realize, "I could have been a better husband, a better father, a better son, a better brother, a better friend."

With autumn comes, the harvest and the pride which comes from a successful effort. You look forward to the harvest. The harvest is the time when it all comes together, and you actually see some rewards for all your labor. You have developed good and loyal patients, some of which have also become friends. But you find that the harvest is work as well, and you begin to find that you don't have the same energy and stamina that you had before. You begin to look forward to putting your feet up and enjoying the fruits of your labor. And because you can no longer cram 20 hours of work into 15 hours, you actually do have to slow down. You can't remember the last time you really felt rested or not on edge, and long to know what that actually feels like.

Winter tells you that your time is short. You're no longer young, and the enjoyment is beginning to be replaced by the frustration of 35 years of a changing environment, and one which no longer rewards time spent with the patient. You need to change, but you don't want to. The changes are not beneficial to your patients, nor to your staff. The rewards are not keeping up with the work and effort that you're putting in. The ground becomes hard, and is no longer plowable. The cold winds blow in, and the snow falls. You get cold, wet and weary. The snow becomes just too much to shovel. The only thing you long for is to be able to put your feet up, a fire in the hearth to keep you warm and family nearby. At that point you know it is over. You say good-bye to all you've known and worked for, and willingly retire to let the younger professionals take your place.

CHAPTER 1

Hospital Rounds

One morning as I drove to the hospital, my mind was racing to process all the information I was given during the night, by the ER physician, about my patient, Viola Warren. She had come into the ER because of severe abdominal pain, which began earlier in the day. They seemed to rule out appendicitis or anything acute, and actually wanted to send her home, but she complained so bitterly about the pain that they decided to keep her overnight for observation.

Viola was an elderly lady in her early 70's who lived alone. She lost her husband 3 years ago, and loneliness was usually her chief complaint. She loved being admitted to the hospital. She saw it as a week at the spa or a 5 star hotel. The nurses and the aides would pamper her, talk to her, give her back rubs and massages, manicure (clip) her toenails, offer her special food and, in general, make her time there most enjoyable. She was able to make new friends, to whom she could tell her medical history, which she loved to do. She was especially fond of the 7 operations she had had and would describe them in minute detail.

When I walked into the ER to see her, she was hooked up to an IV, and was just lying there looking miserable. They had given her some pain meds, so she wasn't writhing as she was when she had come in. I examined her chart, and noted that the exam had been rather precursory. Her blood count and chemistry panel were normal, but she didn't have any X-Ray studies, which surprised me. Hardly anyone leaves the ER dead or alive without catching a few rays. Most patients got the X-Rays done before seeing the physician. I figured that the other 5 patients brought in after a major car accident may have taken the physician's attention away from her.

I closed the curtain around her, and examined her abdomen. It felt like she swallowed a basketball. It was distended and tender to touch. I said to myself, "I guess I'd better do a rectal exam and see what's happening on the other end." That was one exam that neither the doctor nor the patient really wanted or enjoyed. I asked her to roll on her left side, put on a glove with some KY Jelly, and slowly put my index finger into her rectum. It was at that point that a geyser of fecal fluid shot out of her, just missing my shoulder and decorating the curtains and wall with that unmistakably odiferous *eau de merde*, which then filled the entire ER. At the same time Viola exclaimed, "Oh, that feels so much better," I thought, "Oh, this is not good." "They'll kill me for this. I might even get the bill for the cleaning."

But what I said to Viola was, "I just pulled the plug. Your sewer system was backed up. When was the last time you moved your bowels?"

"Oh, I don't know exactly but I've been taking these laxative drinks for the past 4 days and nothing happened."

"Well, Viola, something just happened. I don't think you'll need to take those drinks for a while. Why don't we get you cleaned up and we'll get you out of here."

"Do I have to leave? Can't I stay? Just for a few days anyway?"

"No, Viola. Your insurance won't pay for your stay, and we really need the beds for people that are sick, not just constipated."

"Nobody ever thinks I'm sick," she whined. "Everyone says how good I look. I can't help it if I was born with naturally rosy cheeks. I'm just as sick as everyone else, and no one believes me."

"Viola, I believe, that you believe that you're sick. But just the 2 of us believing that is not going to get you admitted to the hospital. In the pantheon of sickness, yours is not serious enough to warrant being in a hospital. Plus if you do get admitted, the nurse will probably kill you for what you just did to the ER."

"Would they really?"

"No, Viola. I'm just kidding. But they might put you to work cleaning this place up."

I called for a nurse, who when she walked in, looked around and exclaimed, "Oh, $##$. What the hell happened in here?"

"That's about what happened," I said laughing.

"Oh, you think this is funny? Do you know what it's going to take to clean this up?"

"I really had no control over this," I said, trying to shift the blame. "I really would have preferred that this not have happened. But you have to admit, it is rather funny."

"You wouldn't think it was so funny if *you* had to clean it up."

I walked out to discharge Viola with the nurse glaring at me. I proceeded to walk up the stairs continuing to make my rounds, fully expecting a reprimand from the Chief of Staff.

The first stop on my medical rounds was the ICU. I only had one person there, Betty.

Betty was a 60 year old woman, who had smoked heavily her whole life, and refused to quit, even though encouraged to do so on numerous occasions. She ended up in the ICU because she came in with severe hypoxia (low oxygen levels) and difficulty breathing. On her admission, her situation was extremely grave. It seemed that she was on the brink of having to be put on a ventilator, which she didn't want. The big problem was that she might not be able to be taken off the ventilator if her lungs did not improve. But with intensive respiratory therapy, antibiotics and multiple other medications, she managed to turn the corner, and did not need a ventilator after all.

Then two nights ago at about 2 AM, the nurse called saying she was refusing all her treatments, and saying she just wanted to die. So I dragged myself out of bed, drove back to the hospital to talk to her, and tried to determine why, after it appeared she was going to get better, that she now wanted to die. No answer was forth coming other than repeating over and over the fact that she just wanted to die.

At an impasse, I finally called in her family, her husband and her 2 sons, to either say good-bye to her, or try to talk her out of what was perceived to be lunacy.

As they all walked into her room, a scene played out where the oldest son, who came with his wife, both of whom were dressed very nicely and neatly, considering the hour, met her husband and younger son. The younger son came in with unkempt hair, an old jacket, and torn shirt. The brothers hardly acknowledged one another. It turned out the younger son, who lived with the mother and father, was the black sheep of the family. He lived off of the good graces and kindness of his parents, all the while draining them of their financial resources and security.

When Betty's husband, who was extremely hard of hearing, was told the story of what his wife wanted to do, his response was, "Let her do what she wants." The younger son said that his father had trouble hearing, and didn't understand what he was told. To which the father replied, in a very loud voice, "I understand perfectly well what was said, and she should be allowed to do what she wants." This left me and the nursing staff desperately trying to understand this unexpected and bizarre interaction and response.

The younger son then took the lead role in the negotiations with his mother, in trying to coax her into complying with the medical treatment. It seemed he had the biggest stake in this claim. After all if his mother died, who would fix him his meals, wash his clothes, clean the house or give him money. This seemed to lead to some bargaining and deal making. It became apparent that he was doing some things at home which were making his mother's life miserable, including making the house a regular pig sty. As the conversation ensued, it seemed the mother wanted the younger son to get and keep a job, clean up after himself, quit smoking marijuana and stay out of jail. All of which he agreed to, if she would take her treatments.

After he promised her he would change, she then agreed to resume her treatments. The older brother, who was watching this whole conversation in disbelief, exploded. Through gritted teeth he seethed at his mother, "I was told to come down here at 3 o'clock in the morning so that you could have a clean house? This is about dirty laundry and dirty dishes all over the house?" Then taking the volume up a few octaves, he continued, "If you do this to me again, I'll kill you myself." Then he turned to his younger brother, and in a few octaves even higher said, "If you don't straighten yourself out, get a job and become self-supporting, I'll turn you into the cops myself, and I'll make sure you never get out of jail."

As he walked out of the hospital, the nursing staff and I just looked at each other and thought, "Now that was worth the price of admission."

I reviewed Betty's chart, and she seemed to be making good progress since that episode. When I asked how she was doing, she just said fine, and made no reference to the 3 AM confrontation and neither did I. I told her she may be going home in another day or two if she continued to improve.

The next patient was Tony. Tony was the retired postmaster in town. He had another cardiac event, and was once again admitted for chest pain. Tony was very likeable, and had extremely good manners. When he would visit me in the office, he was always dressed impeccably, in a suit coat and tie, dress pants and polished shoes. Everyone else would arrive in whatever clothes they wore for working on the farm, and with manure on their shoes. When he first arrived, I noticed how he was dressed, and trying to be comical, but not wanting to make fun of his clothes, I looked him over, and asked if he was going out on a date, or if he were meeting the President, after the office visit, because it looked as if he were dressed for such an occasion. His response was exemplary of a past generation. He said he was dressed up because he wanted to show me the respect he felt I deserved. "After all you're my doctor."

Tony was Italian and, on his first visit, had to tell an Italian joke. He said, "Do you know why there are so many Italians named Tony? No? It's because when they got on the boat in Italy, they had a sign pinned on their shirts, To New York or ToNY." After that at each visit either he'd tell a joke, or I would tell him one. We got along very well together.

Tony was a combat vet of WWII, and would relate some of his harrowing experiences during the war. His unit was the 28th Infantry Division, which they called "the bloody bucket" because of the insignia on their shoulders. After what he saw, he said the name was appropriate. He was assigned to Patton's 3rd Army for a while, and was in the thick of the fighting. He was convinced that God never left his side. As men were falling all around him, and bullets were whizzing around him, he never got hit. He said it was a miracle. Tony was a very devout Christian believer, and we would talk routinely about his faith, how it got him through the war and how it enabled him to bear the heartache of losing his son at a young age, a heartache he never really got over.

But Tony also had his limits. His daughter, Anna, married Ben, a guy who was not as refined as Tony. Ben would brag about imagined exploits, and would bully his wife and children, but he was really quite kind and considerate with everyone else. One day when Anna was visiting her father, he noticed some bruising on Anna. He asked how she hurt herself, and Anna said she fell off a chair she was standing on. But Tony's grandson, not quite 5, said that "Daddy hit Mommy." That night Tony went over to see Ben. Doing his best Mafia impersonation, he took a gun and put it to Ben's head and told him, "If you ever lay a hand on my daughter again, I'll put a bullet right through your head." That was the last time Anna was bruised. Ben then became a model husband and father. I asked Tony if he'd really shoot Ben. “No, I’d never do that, in fact the gun wasn’t even loaded, but I’m not against making him think I would. Some people just need the right motivation to do the right thing.”

As Tony got older, he started having trouble with his heart. He was proud to hold the University of Massachusetts record for the most cardiac catheterizations ever performed on any one patient. He peaked out at over 15 procedures. At this time cardiac caths and angioplasties were just coming into their own, so I suspected they were using him for practice, to allow all the residents to have experience in doing these procedures. Sometimes he would have an angioplasty, sometimes a stent was put in, but after a while, there was just nothing left for them to do.

During this hospitalization, Tony was once again admitted for chest pain. He was treated conservatively and when I saw him, he was doing better. His chest pain was gone and he was breathing easy again. “Nothing more to do than make sure he was stable and discharge him,” I thought. After a stay in the hospital, Tony always made sure he sent the nurses and those who cared for him a fruit basket, some pastries and flowers to show his gratitude. He was quite the gentleman.

Next stop was the medical floor.

Marilee was a 50 yr. old woman who, after undergoing breast cancer treatment, her doctors thought had been cured. I saw her for her more mundane problems like her high blood pressure and minor illnesses. She came in one day after being told they found she now had metastatic cancer to her liver and bones. She was now looking at treatment with more chemotherapy, and with it, the associated sickening side effects. She had already lost her beautiful red hair. During her routine visits for her blood pressure check, I asked her how she was coping with her treatments, the emotional impact of her diagnosis and whether she had people praying for her and supporting her. She said she did, and that she considered this cancer a blessing from God. Now I had heard cancer called a lot of things, but never a blessing from God. Unable to understand how such a horrific disease could be considered a blessing, I asked her how she considered it to be so.

She related to me that 2 years prior her childless, married daughter was having abdominal pain, and was diagnosed with a tubal pregnancy. During the operation, the surgeon removed the affected tube, cutting it out and eliminating any chance that she would ever get pregnant from that ovary again. While they were operating on her, the surgeon, as surgeons are in the habit of doing, inspected the other ovary. What he saw was a tumor on the other ovary, which required the removal of that entire ovary. Doing this effectively made sure she would never be able to ever have a child, period. To make matters worse, the mass turned out to be an aggressive ovarian cancer, which was usually fatal.

Marilee related that when this occurred she prayed to God that, if it were possible, that her daughter's cancer would be given to her, and for her daughter to be healed. Miraculously the daughter was healed, and even more miraculously, she became pregnant, and had a healthy baby. It was nine months after she said that prayer that she developed her breast cancer.

Marilee was currently in the hospital for the devastating side effects of her cancer treatment. I was always amazed that through all her misery, she never complained. When asked how she was faring, she would always say, "God has been so good to me. He has given me such a great gift. My daughter is alive, and now I have a beautiful grandchild." She would tell this to everyone in the hospital who took care of her.

It was difficult for me to watch her slow demise. I really admired her faith but I didn't fully understand it. Her care was really in the hands of the Oncologist, so I just stopped in to say hello and see how she was faring during her hospitalization.

It was during this hospitalization that her treating doctor noted in her chart that she was terminal and there was no further treatment that could be given, except for palliation of pain.

Marilee was not told this but when I asked how she was doing this time around, she told him, "I'm looking forward to seeing my Lord, who has done great things for me. He has been so good to me."

Not knowing what to say, I just said that I would be praying for her. I wasn't really sure how God answered prayers, but apparently Marilee's prayers were answered. At the time I wasn't sure if that was the prayer I would have prayed or the answer that I would have wanted. But some years afterwards watching someone I love go through cancer treatment, I know that I would have gladly taken her diagnosis and her suffering on myself to save her from it. But we don't get to choose.

These theological questions seemed to come up all the time. And I had never really studied theology very deeply, nor was I raised in a home where these kinds of discussions ever went on. So initially I pushed it to the back of my mind, and figured I had to deal with the here, the now and the practical aspect of taking care of my patients. But as time went on, I realized that these theological questions were more important than what to do about their illnesses. What people thought about the big questions: is there a God, does He care about me, why was I born, what is the meaning of life and what is my purpose determined how they related to others and how they reacted in times of crisis and stress.

If one thinks that we are all just an evolutionary accident, then we are an insignificant cog in the circle of life, and life really has no ultimate meaning. We are here to live, reproduce and die. These people usually put all their hope and trust in their being able to accumulate money, fame or power in order to feel significant and to have the right connections. They chase pleasure and self-indulgence to give their lives meaning.

But if one believes that we were created by a caring and loving God, who wants us to have a close relationship with Him and with others, then we have significance through our relationships with Him and others. By serving Him, our lives have meaning and purpose. These folks place their hope and trust in God and don't need to pursue those things that will get someone into trouble in life. They have an inner strength to meet life in the times of crisis. Because of this, I began to ask my patients about their thoughts about God and life during their visits. Some loved to talk about it and welcomed the conversation. Others felt uncomfortable and thought it strange that their doctor would ask about such personal details, although talking about the intimate details about their sex life, their toilet life or their marital life didn't seem to bother them. And others would reject the questions or even become combative, and would let me know it was none of my business.

This was the life I had chosen, sight unseen. It certainly wasn't what I was expecting when I was in high school thinking about "what do I want to be when I grow up?"

Chapter 2

How did I end up here??

In 1976 I had finished my residency in Family Medicine in Minnesota, and wanted a family friendly and old fashioned town in which to practice.

I planned to plant my practice in rural Vermont. It seemed ideal, as I had envisioned it—a small town, of good and kindly people in a setting like a Norman Rockwell painting. I was encouraged to go to Vermont by the director of our residency, who was from Vermont, and had been a family practitioner for many years before changing career paths. He said he had a friend, an older doc, in small town Vermont, who was looking for an associate to take over his practice before he retired. It seemed perfect—the mountain backdrop, the church on the village green, the clean air, the blazing colors of the leaves in the fall, the blanket of snow in the winter, the greens and flowers of the spring and summer.

I thought I was following my dream, but it was a dream not based in any reality. Certainly it was not based on anything I had ever known or experienced. I was born in Brooklyn, New York. Not quite the rural area where we had settled to practice. The city had small communities, but they were measured in blocks, not miles. It was also very diverse. Walking 10 blocks might take you from the Irish neighborhood, through the Italian neighborhood, past the German neighborhood and into the Jewish neighborhood. The only neighborhood you didn't go through was the rich neighborhood, because there weren't any where we lived. In a few short blocks one could pass by the German butcher, the German bakery, the Jewish delicatessen, an Italian pastry shop, a dry cleaner, a shoemaker, a local grocery, a few pubs (or bars as they were known) and a few candy and newspaper stores, which also had soda fountains where you could get ice cream floats or egg cream sodas. Going into each of these shops, one's memory was impressed more by the distinctive smell rather than by the physical appearance. A counter, display and advertising posters were all present in each. But the smell of corned beef, apple strudel, cannoli, bagels, bologna or beer was how they were really identified. You could be blind and know exactly which store you had stepped into.

I remember the Rheingold beer ads most of all. This beer was a New York beer, started by a German family in 1883. In the 1950's Rheingold beer would have an election, in October, for a young woman, who would be crowned Miss Rheingold for the next year. She would then be the face of the beer and used in all the advertisements for that year. The winner was as anticipated as the mayoral election each year, and likely had more people voting in it. Where we grew up, everyone was a Democrat so the local political elections were never in any doubt. If you didn't vote the right way, someone would knock on your door and give you a reminder that your job was dependent on the right person being elected. Enough said. Rheingold had a great jingle, which was set to the tune of "Colonel Bogey March" ("The Bridge over the River Kwai" theme song). Sixty years later, the catchy tune still stands the test of time.

The buildings were tenements with brick fronts and a varying number of steps going up to the front doors. There were usually 3 apartments per building—ground floor, 2nd floor and top floor—and no elevators. Groceries etc. were all carried up the stairs. Low picket fences separated the building and its ground floor windows from the pedestrians walking the street, thus giving each building a "front yard," so to speak, where one could place a chair, and sit and watch the goings on in the neighborhood. There was no need for street cameras. The older women of the neighborhood were almost always watching, either from the windows or the front yards. Today these same buildings sell for millions of dollars.

Most activities in the good weather were happening outside. Sitting on the steps, the inhabitants would talk to neighbors, eat snacks and keep track of the kids, who would be playing stick ball, hopscotch or hide and seek in the streets. The kids would sound the alarm of "Car," which was the signal to get on the sidewalk, each time a car wanted to drive down the street. In the summer, everyone would swelter, as there was no air-conditioning. Men walking around in short sleeve or no sleeve undershirts would have sweat glisten on their necks and shoulders. Women would wear sun dresses, and stay near a fan. In the winter, they dressed in layers, and took showers or baths less frequently, as there was usually a chill in the apartment with landlords trying to reduce heating costs.

When all the windows were open, one could walk down the street, take in the smells and identify what was cooking in each apartment, so you would know what everybody was having for dinner that night. Any arguments amongst family members or neighbors, could also be clearly heard outside the buildings. There were no secrets that were able to be hidden in that environment. We all knew when the wooden spoon was used to punish child law breakers in the homes as well.

In the summer, what one most likely heard when walking by the apartments was a baseball game. The Brooklyn Dodgers, who played in Ebbets Field in Brooklyn, and the New York Yankees, who played in Yankee Stadium in the Bronx, were fierce rivals, and the neighborhood was split into Yankee and Dodger camps. The New York Giants, who played in the Polo Grounds in upper Manhattan, was a third NY team, but I never knew anyone who rooted for the Giants. The voices of the announcers of the games were as well known as the US presidents: Red Barber and Vin Scully announcing the Dodgers, Mel Allen and Phil Rizzuto for the Yankees.

As a kid growing up in a neighborhood where all the men were veterans of World War II, and being inundated with movies about the war, I always expected to join the military. If someone asked me what I wanted to be when I grew up at age 7, I would say a soldier.

Walking or subway was how most people got around. If a family had a car, the man used it to get to work. I only knew a few women who worked growing up. One had lost her husband in the war and another worked as a secretary.

When I was 7 years old, my parents moved to Queens. That was the country for us. Houses were separate from each other, and grass grew in front and back as well as a tree or two. In Queens we played baseball in the highway cloverleaf that had a grassy area. Luckily only one time did the ball go sailing out into the highway and was hit by a car, which caused us all to run.

What I knew of medical practice growing up came from visits to our family doctor. And that only came about for something serious—strep throat, ear infections, stitches or operations. Almost every kid had his tonsils out by the time he was 12. Childhood diseases spread throughout the neighborhood, like a wild fire in a forest. Chicken pox, measles, mumps, German measles and whooping cough all made the rounds to each household. The scariest epidemic was the summer polio epidemic, which could cause paralysis and death. Going to the doctor for a well child visit was unheard of, and each visit usually ended up with a shot of penicillin or tetanus. As far as I knew, to be a doctor, all you had to know was how to stitch a laceration, give a shot and do a tonsillectomy.

Of course there were always the doctor themed TV shows, like "Ben Casey," "Dr. Kildare" and "Marcus Welby, MD," in the late1950's and early 60's that made medicine seem interesting, exciting and glamourous. So while in high school, the time came to apply to colleges, and my guidance counselor asked me what I wanted to do. I thought, "I want to get out of New York. I want to live where the air is clear and the people are friendly. I want the quiet of a country road without all the honking of horns, sirens and people yelling at one another. I want my kids to be able to play baseball on a baseball field, not on an interstate highway." But I said, "I think I'd like to be a psychiatrist," because at that time there was a popular TV show on about psychiatrists. What I didn't pick up on was the fact that these psychiatrists lived in a city. The guidance counselor never asked me why psychiatry, what I knew about psychiatry, what I was interested in or what my aptitude tests indicated I should study. He simply said, "Oh, that's a big one. You have to go to medical school first, and then go to study psychiatry." "Oh, OK. So I'll go to medical school." Now my guidance counselor could have just as well told me, I'd have to go live on Mars. I had just as much knowledge about going to Mars as I had about going to college, or medical school for that matter. But I was willing to put up with any inconvenience, bear any burden or suffer any pain to be able to leave the city.

Being the first one in my family to go to college, I received no practical advice about what college was all about, and didn't really know what to expect. Almost all the adults in the neighborhood were without college educations, so there was no information coming from outside the family either. College life, I thought, was what you saw in movies, not what anyone had actually experienced. Of course in the movies, one never saw anyone actually studying in college. There were only the hijinks, the fun times and the boy-girl interactions. So trying to find out what college and medical practice were all about by watching TV and movies was like trying to figure out what being a policeman was like by watching the Andy Griffith show.

As it turned out, life in college was a lot like living on Mars for me. I lived in a dorm with 2 roommates, one who would suddenly jump up and start doing jumping jacks, and the other who would talk in his sleep. The 3 guys next door were an odd lot also. At 10 PM every night one would open the window and yell out, "It's Red Sox baseball," for no good reason. One of his roommates, when asked a question, would start to recite Beowulf in Old English, and the other would sleep in a sleeping bag on the floor so he didn't have to make his bed. Now it wasn't as if I was used to having a room of my own, because I had to share a bedroom with my brother at home. But I never before had to live with people, who may have been truly certifiable. Maybe this would be good experience for someone going into psychiatry, I didn't know.

There was enforced study and quiet time between 7-10 PM each night, if there were classes the next day. Between 10-11 PM pandemonium would break out, and then it was enforced lights out at 11 PM. But you could go to a study hall, which was open all night and which I used a lot, to study. You didn't go to the study hall for comfort. It was very monastic and furnished with long wooden tables and hard, straight back chairs. The basic philosophy of the school was if the conditions were comfortable, you weren't studying hard enough.

The school mainly drew its students from NY, CT, MA and RI, making it very regional. Those from CT, MA and RI would go home every weekend on Friday afternoon and return Sunday night, leaving those from NY, with no cars or transportation, to entertain themselves at an all-male college. The usual entertainment was devising practical jokes to play on other students, the most hilarious having to do with water, grease or flash bulbs in a pitch black room. One holiday weekend when the entire dorm seemed empty, those of us left were all confined to quarters after a particularly loud sink-ball game (a modification on basketball using empty milk cartons and the sink in the room) which had annoyed the resident priest living on the same floor. Justice was meted out in a very capricious manner.

The college was run by the Order of Dominicans, the very same order that also ran the Inquisition during the Middle Ages. It was during that time period that they perfected methods of torturing heretics, methods which were assiduously passed down the generations to the priests running this college. It wasn't the physical torture that was feared, it was the psychological torture that broke most, at this school.

The first day of classes in college, I found out that the head of the pre-med department had as his goal to fail the entire class. He said it had never been done, but this class had great potential for that accomplishment. He was constantly playing the hidden assignment game. He'd assign the class to read chapters 1-5 in the book, and then give the test on chapters 6-10. When everyone failed the test, it was pointed out to him that he had assigned chapters 1-5, but we were tested on chapters 6-10. His response was, "Well you should have known better." Or he would ask questions on obscure footnotes. I thought that this guy's goal should have been to avoid assassination.

One priest who was an outlier taught the theology course. It was supposed to teach us how to be good Catholics. This guy's course taught us all religions were the same and not really based in reality. After taking that course, most students left the Catholic Church. His last year of teaching was my year. After the course was over, he left the church and became a Buddhist. This made everyone wonder how the college administration could let this kind of teaching go on at a supposed Roman Catholic institution. But then it was discovered that the president of the college had his own issues with the "one true faith" as well. He was discovered to have a girlfriend. After she became pregnant, he left the order and the college, and married her.

One of the only good things that happened while going to college was getting back to seeing Maria. We knew each other before, as we had gone to the same elementary school, and were in the same class. We were friends in high school, but really didn't start dating until we were in college. I had fallen in love with Maria in high school—her sparkling blue eyes, her warm smile and her strawberry blonde hair—but could never seem to get her to go on more than one date. No other girl ever interested me. After high school we got reacquainted and I wooed her by making her think that I actually knew what I was going to do, and was kind and witty, and compassionate. I knew I was none of these and not what she deserved, but for her I would try to change.

After her family moved to New Jersey, it necessitated an hour long trip from my house to hers in order to see her when I was home from college. The Cross Bronx Expressway and the George Washington Bridge became very familiar territory. It was a highway that was littered with garbage, broken glass, partially stripped abandoned cars and burning tires, and was patrolled by gangsters. If you got lost or stuck on that road, you and your car would probably never be seen again. I had always heard the joke that people in NY were always depressed because they knew the light at the end of the tunnel was NJ, but this part of NY would not be called a garden state either.

CHAPTER 3

Medical School

During medical school, psychiatry became less attractive. It was probably the rotation I had in the ward for the criminally insane that put me off. These patients not only heard voices, but those voices told them to kill you. The really scary part of that rotation was going out to your car. The same people walking the streets were also hearing voices telling them to rob, maim and pummel you into a mass of contusions and abrasions. The whole area was a mental patient rich environment.

When doing my psychiatric rotation, I talked to the psychiatric residents and asked them why they chose to go into psychiatry. The answers I got were amusing. One said that he was finding that all his patients were crazy so he might as well try to get to the root of their problem. Another said he didn't really want to deal with really sick people, another so he could understand his crazy family better, and another saw the same program I saw on TV and thought psychiatry was sitting at a nice oak desk in a beautifully designed office, smoking a pipe and listening to people's problems, but never really having to cure anyone. It was always, "OK, I'll see you again next week," and away they would go. No hassle about having to find new patients or finding the cure. Of course if they did actually cure the patient, that would mean they wouldn't have to come back next week and that income source would be over, and so would their paycheck. There was a certain amount of job security involved in that profession.

After my experiences in medical school, I became more interested in becoming a small town, Marcus Welby type of doctor (from the TV show), and decided to go into family medicine. But again, I really had no idea what small town medicine was all about, having never really lived in one. I had no idea what real practice entailed, and certainly didn't realize it entailed running a business. So going to a rural area would be just as much of an adventure in all things new for me as it was for my patients, who I would meet for the first time.

It was during med school that Maria and I got married. It was supposed to be a traditional wedding in the church we both grew up in. Unfortunately, neither my family nor Maria's family lived near or went to that church any longer. But after the church we were supposed to get married in released us in return for 2 future weddings and 3 draft picks, we got permission to marry in our former church.

The wedding site was a bit of a logistical nightmare, as it was between the two families, but near neither. Maria's family in NJ decided to rent a bus and take all the family and friends together, and that way no one would have to worry about drinking and driving. When the wedding time arrived, the bride, the bride's father, the groom and the groom's family were all there. However the bride's mother was nowhere to be found. It turned out that the bride's mother was on a bus lost somewhere in the middle of Manhattan. Fortunately for them, someone had stocked the bus with all sorts of liquor and lots of it. The attitude of those on the bus was basically, "We don't care if we never get there. We're having a great time on the bus." To put it succinctly, they were in no hurry to get to the church on time.

Unfortunately, Father John wanted to get the wedding started because this wedding was beginning to run into other events that were supposed to take place at the church that afternoon and evening, and he needed the church emptied of the wedding for those events to take place. Maria, not wanting to get married without her mother present, hid in the ladies room so no one could get to her. After about an hour and a half, and at about the same time Father John was drawing up the papers of excommunication for all of us, the wayward bus from NJ arrived.

As they all rolled into the church, it was obvious that the party had started without those who were waiting at the church. The wedding then went off without a hitch, except for when it came to the reception of Communion. Some of the NJ guests, who when they were offered communion, said they didn't need any wine from Father John, because they had better stuff of their own, and one lady who thought the chalice was all for her, attempted to drain it before giving it back to Father John. After the marriage, at the same time he had us sign the marriage certificates, Father John had Maria and I sign papers promising under pain of excommunication, in effect, that no one from either family would ever get married in his church again.

Marriage seems to be less popular than it once was. Couples are not getting married as often as they used to. They have no problem with living together, and even having kids together, but marriage doesn't seem to be as attractive as a no or low commitment relationship. People tend not to get married because a) they don't need a legal paper to prove that they love one another, b) don't want to have to get divorced if they break up - just walk away, no fuss no muss, c) don't want that legally binding commitment straining their relationship or d) all of the above.

Some will say that they're waiting to get married until they have enough money for the wedding they want. But what they're really saying is that they want an extravagant party. The wedding itself is not much more expensive than a movie and dinner.

Church weddings are also becoming a thing of the past. Now you need to go to a wedding venue which provides, the place - usually with a gazebo or outdoor garden - the person officiating, the party, the band and the food all at the same place. It's one stop shopping. Or even better, a destination wedding, where all your guests need to book plane reservations and meet at some exotic or, what is assumed to be, romantic hideaway. Weddings are no longer sacred. They no longer begin with "We are gathered here in the sight of God and His church to witness the union of this man and this woman in holy matrimony." God is no longer invited. God is no longer is considered essential and need not be involved. No longer do those getting married promise to "have and to hold, from this day forward, for better or worse, for richer, for poorer, in sickness and in health, to love and to cherish, till death do us part." Now everyone makes up their own vows, which basically says, "I promise to love you until I don't as long as the sun continues to shine."

Once a man went up to his pastor and said that his marriage was falling apart and wanted to get a divorce. He told the pastor, "This is worse than I ever imagined." The pastor told him, "Well, you promised you'd hold on to her for better or worse. You got worse. Work it out."

But marriage is so much more. It is not just living or hanging out with your "best friend." It is being joined together so closely that the two become one. When one gets married, one shares not only experiences, but also a life. You live in the same house, sleep in the same bed, eat the same food, and go to the same weddings and baptisms. You share the same relatives, the same bank account, the same car and the same pets. And most importantly, you share the same children. You share the same sorrows and the same joys. And all these things that you share basically create the effect of living the same life. The more years that go by, the closer their bond and the greater their love grows. When done right, marriage, like fine wine, gets better with age.

One usually thinks of marriage when they are "young and in love." But as it turns out, one does not really know what love is all about until one is married for 40-50 years.

Residency

After med school I went to Minnesota for a family practice residency. The reason I went there, rather than, say, California or Florida, was that I wanted to experience bone-chilling cold weather for 7 months out of the year. Plus the residency had a program where the residents could spend 1 or 2 months at a clinic in Frostbite Falls, on the boundary waters, only reachable by snowmobile in the winter and by canoe in the summer. The temperature in the winter was usually around 40 below zero, and in the 2 days of summer the mosquitoes come out in swarms, and could drain the blood out of a moose and kill it in 60 seconds. You could try insect repellent, but that just seemed to attract them. Who could pass up that kind of experience?

In the winter with below zero temps, it snowed just about every day. With that kind of winter, one would think that the summers would be delightful. If one did, one would be wrong. It was generally about 100 degrees all summer, or what there was of it.

It was in Minnesota that I saw hospitals, for the first time that looked like 5 star hotels, and not a stripped down version of a Motel 6 or the dungeon of Frankenstein. Some of the docs were pretty amazing too. After admitting a patient, the residents would discuss the case amongst themselves, try to come up with a working diagnosis and present it to the preceptor. One of our preceptors, Dr. Fred Walker, would then listen to the resident's presentation of a particularly complicated case with all the possibilities given, and then Fred would say, "He's got ________." And sure enough he did. It was uncanny.

Fred wanted me to practice in Minnesota when I finished my residency, but I had other ideas. I really wanted to live in New England. When Fred asked why New England, I said I like it because it's historic, scenic and quaint. Fred then told me, "Don't choose where you want to live by the geography. There's more to living in a place than hills and valleys, mountains and lakes." No truer words were ever spoken. Who you live with is far more important than where you live. The most beautiful town could be inhabited by serial killers or ax murderers - or more likely by mean, greedy, envious and hate filled people. But I had to test this out to see for myself.

Across the hall from the apartment we lived in, were Beth and Bob from Slippery Rock, Pennsylvania. Bob worked for American Motors

Auto Company, best known for the Gremlin, the Pacer, the Javelin and the Nash-Rambler. The company went out of business in 1988, which was almost inevitable given its car lineup.

Beth was a high school math and science teacher, and although she was very petite, she could give a 6'4" 300 lb. high school senior a look that would paralyze him. It was known around the school as "the look of death." She was a lot like a bobcat. Everyone thinks they can take it on, and beat it in a fight, but nobody tries.

CHAPTER 4

In Vermont I found the ground for planting a practice as hard as the granite mountains. The good and kindly people were also hard as granite. They were content with a pick-up truck or 4 wheel drive vehicle, a rifle and a 6 pack of beer. They lived off the land with whatever they could hunt, fish or farm out of it. They were land rich and bank account poor.

When I was in VT, it was a very rural state, known for milk, cheese, maple syrup, granite and teddy bears. It was run by rock ribbed Republicans, who really did believe that a penny saved was a penny earned. I imagine that these folks didn't know what hit them after the progressives and socialists moved in, and took over their government. Now they're known for being the only state to have a socialist senator, environmentally safe manure and rapidly declining farms. Dairy farms have declined from 11,000 to 1,000 over the past 50 years. Just a guess on my part but I'll bet that marijuana farmers have increased, as there are currently no governmental regulations on the growth, storage or production, unlike the poor dairy farmer.

It takes a special type of person to live in a climate with 3 seasons of winter and 4 weeks of rough sledding. They even had a season that the rest of the country did not. It was called mud season. Now if you're like me, who was not brought up in the rural northeast, when you hear mud, you don't really make much of it. After all, all our streets were paved. How bad could it be? Well, when you've got dirt roads, the mud can be quite formidable. There were tales of tow trucks having to be called out to pull a 4 wheel drive vehicle, whose driver thought he could go anywhere on the planet, out of mud that was over its axles. Some farmers would tell of mud so bad they'd lose whole cows just trying to cross a field. And I was not one to dispute them. Now that a lot of their roads are paved, they can roll mud season into the 4 weeks of rough sledding season.

I took over the office practice of another doc, who went back to do a residency. He in turn had taken the practice over from another doc, who also didn't last there long. There was no pharmacy in town, so if you wanted a prescription filled, one had to take the ride to Brattleboro. So to alleviate that problem the docs had large jugs of pills of various medications, high blood pressure meds, diabetes meds, antibiotics, pain meds, some heart meds (like Digoxin) and diuretics, but the majority were filled with anti-anxiety and sleeping pills. These were the main meds that were prescribed. This was before pills were available to treat high cholesterol, heart disease and pulmonary disease. We also considered diabetes controlled if there was no sugar in the urine and cholesterol controlled if it was below 300, so these diagnoses were much less common then.

Renting an office above us was a dentist, who had just gotten out of the military and wanted to move back to Vermont. I thought he was a nice guy and very helpful. He'd let me borrow some of his dental instruments if I needed to work on a patient. Unfortunately his wife had no love of Vermont and his practice and his marriage failed. She told him if he wanted a house out in the woods, he could, but she wasn't going to be in it.

I got to the office every day and put out the Bennington flag, which was my way of letting people know that "the doctor was in." I would then see a few patients in the morning, broke for lunch, when I walked to the post office to pick up our mail, then would go back and see a few patients in the afternoon, and leave about 5 PM.

Barbara, my nurse, receptionist, assistant and office manager, was smart and one of the hardest working and nicest persons I ever had the pleasure to come upon. I inherited her from the previous doc. She managed the inventory and supplies, sent out the bills, answered the phone, made appointments, and assisted me, sometimes all at the same time. But no matter how we scrimped to cut expenses, the income was not coming in. This situation existed even in light of the fact that the hospital, which owned the office, didn't charge me for rent and provided basic office supplies like toilet paper and light bulbs.

Barbara had a wonderful family, who were kind and welcoming. They made maple syrup in the spring, farmed and cut wood in the summer, hunted and cut wood in the fall and tried to keep warm in the winter. These were hard working people. I believe most of the older Vermonters were like this before the liberal and drug addled moved in.

In Vermont I had to cover the ER at night, and unfortunately that was when I saw the majority of my patients for the day. There were always the intoxicated teenaged boys, who somehow got into some accident that required stitches or a cast or both, usually the result of a "double dog dare" during an intoxicated binge. I'd also see the emergency sore throat or earache which couldn't be seen during regular office hours for one reason or another, and the out of towners. They were passing through, and wanted to "get checked out" before they hit the ski slopes or start their vacation.

My fee for an office visit was usually $5-$7, and when I had to go in for an ER visit, I'd charge $10. Unfortunately, it really didn't matter what I charged. The old Vermonters may have wanted to pay, but didn't have the money to pay, and the tourists from the liberal states of Connecticut and Massachusetts didn't pay you, because, I reckon, they didn't think they should have to. I guess this was the beginning of the "healthcare is a right and I shouldn't have to pay for it" movement. There were many false names and addresses as well as phony insurance information given to the person registering these folks. No ID's were required, and there was no way to check the validity of any information given. Once in a while I'd receive some eggs or some other food for payment from my Vermont patients, but unfortunately, when my bills came in, my creditors were not interested in bartering. They wanted cash, gold, silver, diamonds, precious metals, valuable jewelry or other hard currency.

The hospital I worked at was labor intensive. All we had for diagnostics was blood analysis, which was sent out to a lab, with the results being available in 2-3 days, and plain X-Rays. But there were no X-Ray techs and no staff other than a nurse, who not only covered the ER but also the inpatients. If an X-Ray was required, I had to take it, develop it and read it. And in those days X-Rays were developed in a dark room with a red light and solutions in which to place the negatives in order to develop them.

They also installed a 2 way radio in my car so the ER could call me if I wasn't in the office or at home within reach of a telephone. Some days I would be driving home from the office when they would call and say I needed to see someone in the ER. And that would be the end of dinner and any family time.

The labor and delivery was on the 2nd floor and since there were no elevators in the building, the women, while in labor, had to climb up a very steep, long and narrow staircase in order to get there. There was no anesthesia available and no specialists to call if one needed help with a difficult delivery or to do a Caesarian section. I could do forceps deliveries very well, but I wasn't trained to do C-Sections alone. I would only assist. Because of this, one time I had to call an ambulance for a woman who was having trouble delivering. The good news was they would take her to Brattleboro, where those facilities were available. The bad news was it was a 45 minute ride and a lot could happen on route. They also had to get her down that same staircase that she had climbed up. Putting a pregnant woman, in labor, on a stretcher, and carrying her down a stairway at a 45 degree angle, usually did not end well.

Once I had an older guy, who had an accident, broke his ankle and really needed an orthopedist to put some pins in. When I told him he needed to be taken to Brattleboro, he said to me, "just patch me up the best you can, Doc. I'm sure it'll be OK." So I set it, put a cast on it and had him non-weight bearing for 8-10 weeks, and sure enough, it healed.

Before long it became clear that this practice was not going to work out. I slowly found out that I had a number of circumstances that were working against my establishing a thriving practice. One was the fact that I was a "flatlander," i.e., a non-Vermonter. They were very untrusting of "visitors who stayed." Once I had a conversation with a patient, and told him that my wife was going to have a baby. I said that my child would be a Vermonter. To which he said to me, "Just because the kittens come out of the oven, don't make 'em muffins." It seemed like you weren't really to be trusted until your grandfather was buried in the local cemetery.

The second problem was that this town and this practice were known for burning through doctors. The docs would come, set up a practice then leave. So the general consensus of the population was, "don't bother to establish yourself with that doctor. He'll probably be leaving soon. Stick with someone you know will stay here."

Which brings me to the third problem: The old doc, who wanted an associate so he could pass his practice on to him, had no intention of retiring. He only wanted someone to take over for him when he wanted to take some time off. And he did not want to share his patients with anyone, new or old. If I saw one of his patients when he was away, he'd be sure to tell them that they were expected to see him for their next visit, not me. He would insinuate that I might not be there for their next visit, to not discourage them from keeping him as their doctor. Since he was personal friends with the governor of the state and had a great deal of influence in the town, his word carried a lot of weight.

The fourth problem was that my wife was getting cabin fever. We only had one car that did not do well on snowy roads, so she was stuck in a small house with 2 children under the age of 3 and one on the way. I was tired and irritable and didn't treat her as kindly as I should have, when I finally got home. This did not make her time in Vermont enjoyable at all. It was more like living in the movie, *The Shining*. I think she half expected me to come home one night with an axe and say the famous line, "Here's Johnny!"

The last problem I was dealing with was financial. Having a wife, two children and one on the way made finances an issue. We were just about able to make ends meet because we had very little in the way of expenses. We had no rent to pay. In the summer we lived in the old doc's house in the center of town for free, while he moved to his "cabin" on top of the mountain. Come fall, we lived in another lady's house when she left to go to Florida for the winter—winter being October to June. We could not afford to buy a house, let alone rent one. We looked at some property but as soon as they found out it was a doctor from Connecticut looking, the price tripled. Not that I hold it against someone for trying to make a profit. I am a capitalist. But $250,000 for an acre on the side of a mountain, without a house, water, electric or road, seemed to be a bit over the top given the economy, especially when the going price for everyone else was less than $1,000.

Our financial situation was so poor that when we went to buy a 4 wheel drive vehicle, the car salesman told me he couldn't sell me one without a cosigner because I was such a loan risk. They said I didn't make enough money to pay the loan off. I made more money during my internship at $800/month, than I did in this practice. However, we needed a 4 wheel drive car. In the winter you couldn't get around without one. We had gone up there with a Chrysler Scamp, a back wheel drive car that would slide sideways and skid all over the roads.

In a move of desperation, I sent out a letter to each of my patients who had an account balance. It gave an account of the services rendered and what was owed me. I told them if they couldn't pay the whole amount to just cross out the number, and put in any amount they felt they could pay, or whatever they thought would be fair. I would then accept this as payment in full. From that letter writing campaign I got exactly zero dollars.

I loved the mountains and the farms and would have loved to have stayed. The problem was my wife. While Maria liked living in the country, she also liked being able to pay her bills. If a bill came in, she paid it immediately, and had the check in the mail the next day.

When she was unable to get the check in the mail the following day, she was unhappy. Luckily for me, Maria lived very simply, and managed the household budget frugally. She wasn't one for jewelry or expensive clothes. She was able to sew the children's clothes from scraps of fabric she would pick up on sale, and we never ate out, nor did we take vacations. Unluckily for me, even with these measures, our savings would be depleted in 4-6 weeks.

To live in Vermont was my dream and I didn't want to give up on it, but my wife gave me an ultimatum. She was leaving and taking the kids. I could stay if I wanted to or I could come with her. Since we were pretty much broke, and needing loans, we left. So feeling like a failure, I packed up my family and we moved from small town Vermont to small town rural Connecticut. I figured if I could endure the Cross Bronx Expressway for my wife, I surely could endure leaving Vermont. Parting from her would have been too much for me to bear.

CHAPTER 5

The Early Years

As I said before, I really didn't know what life in a small town would be like, and I certainly didn't know what practicing medicine would be like. All the "big city" problems that we had to deal with in medical school and residency, I thought would be a thing of the past after moving to the idyllic small town atmosphere of dear hearts and gentle church going people. Surely there would be accidents and illnesses, but gone would be the problems of drug use, alcoholism, addiction, severe depression (after all, who could be sad living in such a place) and severe mental illness. It would be like Nirvana. I had seen a practice I thought was like that when I was in medical school.

I did a short term clerkship in a small town in CT with a family doctor in medical school. He would spend the mornings leisurely visiting with patients in the small town hospital, where almost all were there to have tests or X-Rays. He would then go to his office in the afternoon and see very pleasant patients and would prescribe meds for their high blood pressure, take care of sore throats or earaches, suture a laceration or two and generally have a peaceful and enjoyable day.

On the weekend, he would attend the local prep school football game, where he acted as team physician, spend the rest of the time with his family and of course go to church on Sunday morning. So with this as the ideal, I left Vermont and headed to CT.

The Eastern Connecticut towns had very interesting demographics. Each had its own character. Bedford, primarily, was divided into Bedford Hill, where the professionals lived along with some of the old families who'd lived there for centuries, and the Northwick section with the old mills and the housing for the mill workers. These folks were generally ethnic: French Canadian, Polish and some Italian and German who were the sons and daughters of the original mill workers.

Bainbridge was primarily a mill town, again with a lot of French Canadians, while East Bainbridge was the "nice" part of town with the old houses and more well-to-do residents.

Roxbury was primarily an agricultural area with lots of farms and had been settled by Yankees and Swedes. Roxbury also had its hill with the old families, and where a private academy resided.

Richmond was the "elite" town. It had the private prep school with all the teachers, professors, professionals and moneyed folks.

Finally, Westford was rural and very Yankee in character.

In Vermont I had to cover the ER. But fortunately soon after I arrived in Bedford, the hospital hired some ER docs to work the nights and weekends. Emergency room physicians were usually drawn to the field by the regular hours, as well as by the reliable and usually higher payment for their services. The hours of boredom followed by minutes of sheer pandemonium and panic was the price paid for that. The part time ER docs were usually older, experienced docs who wanted out of the grueling hours for little pay routine, or were residents looking to supplement their sparse residency pay.

Although most people died at home at that time, the hospital was quickly becoming the location of choice to depart for the next life. More than once, elderly patients would be wheeled into the ER screaming and yelling that they didn't want to be brought to the hospital, because they knew that people, who went to the hospital, died there. Telling these folks that they needed to go to the hospital was more of a death sentence to them than telling them they had cancer. So the ER was becoming a confusing place. People were being seen who had a treatable problem as well as those taking their last breaths, or taking no breaths. Since no family member ever wanted to decide that a loved one was dead, the ER doc and staff were the designated deciders. Not even the ambulance personnel were allowed to say, “This person doesn’t need an ER and a doctor. They need an undertaker.”

CHAPTER 6

The Doctors

After hospital rounds, some of the docs dropped by the doctors' lounge. There were always coffee, donuts and bagels available, along with a variety of conversations. The conversation groups usually broke down into the sports group talking usually about football or baseball depending on the season, the political group arguing over political and public policy issues and the financial group analyzing the stock market's ups and downs and where to invest. There was also the food group comparing the best restaurants in the surrounding area, as well as the travel and vacation group discussing the best travel deals or the best places to go. Then there was the pot luck group, where the conversation could be about anything, including actually comparing and determining the best medical treatments.

Generally I drifted between groups, depending on the conversation. I didn't bet on sports, and while interested, I just wasn't in the same league as the sports group. My political views would isolate me in that group of social engineers. There is no class of people who think they know what the general public and society need best like physicians. If they ruled the world, there would be peace, love, prosperity... and totalitarianism. I didn't understand the financial group, so I'd spend most of my time with the vacation and food groups. Not that we took vacations, but I would live vicariously through those who did, and maybe find some good places to eat, if we ever were able to get out.

My vacations in those days usually involved attending medical educational conferences someplace where I could take my family. I would be locked in a dark room without windows, while the family would take the "family tours" to see the local places of interest. Through these trips, we got to see a rodeo in Dallas, a Mardi Gras in the Superdome in New Orleans, a Kansas City barbeque, Disney Land and Universal Studios for an evening. My family got to see the White House, Capitol building, Fort McHenry and DC museums.

The best thing about going to the doctor's lounge, though, was getting to know the doctors I practiced with. I got to see who was ethical, who was hard working, who was smart, who I could count on to be there for me and who were greedy, jealous and not to be trusted.

Every new doctor who came into town met Dr. Stone and heard "the speech." Dr. Stone told them that the best doctors had the biggest mortgages, meaning of course that they'd have to work night and day to pay it off. When I first started my practice in Bainbridge, I didn't have the biggest mortgage, but the interest rate on the business loans for equipment etc. was about 25%, thanks to the state of our economy under President Jimmy Carter, and I wanted to get that paid off as soon as possible.

This went along with his second bit of advice: "In order to be a successful doctor, you need 4 attributes: availability, affordability, affability and some ability." He was asked, "What if you have the best ability but no availability, no affordability and no affability? What does that make you?" "A specialist" was his answer.

Dr. Stone also believed that, to be a really good doctor, one had to sacrifice everything on the altar of medicine—including your time and your family. One time when a severe snow storm was predicted to hit the town, he announced that he was volunteering to stay at the hospital "until the crisis was over," in case docs couldn't get through the roads to tend to "the sick and wounded." It was all very dramatic and worthy of at least an honorable mention for nobility. I, on the other hand, being the "new breed" of doctor, who couldn't hold a candle to the "old guard," said (to myself), "What are you nuts?" But to Dr. Stone, I responded, "I'm going home to make sure my family will be safe. I'll be back when I know they'll be OK." Oh, the looks of disdain coming from the old guard were enough to wilt the roses in summer. "They just don't make 'em like they used to" was all they could say, while they shook their collective heads in disbelief. As it turned out, the weatherman, as usual, exaggerated the severity of the storm. The townsfolk really didn't have to gather enough food and water to last the rest of the winter, fill their bathtubs with water and their cars with gas and write letters to their loved ones with updates to their last will and testament. But we did lose electricity for 5 hours. And that was only because a suicidal squirrel got into the transformer and chewed the wires. But the drama that played out in the hospital was memorable.

Another interesting doc, who was the opposite of Dr. Stone, was a family doc who began his practice just a little after Dr. Stone. This new doctor had a good natured, care-free attitude toward work and life. He was never happier than when he was fishing, which he did at every given opportunity. He could figure out more ways of getting out of work than anyone I ever knew. In fact, let's just refer to him by his nickname, Barnacle Bill or Dr. Bill. When I first came to town, I was in a call coverage arrangement with Dr. Bill, who could go a whole weekend and never see one of my patients. The patients would call with a problem, and he would treat them, often times very adequately, without ever seeing them. If they called at night, or if they couldn't get to a pharmacy, he'd go through "the list," meaning he would ask them to inventory their medicine cabinet. Did they have cold preparations, aspirin or cough syrup? If they came up empty, he would start on the pantry. "Do you have grape jelly? Apple cider vinegar? Strawberry jam? ...Great! Take a teaspoon of strawberry jam every 4 hours, and see your regular doctor first thing in the morning." Of course, though, I already had a whole bunch of patients scheduled for the following morning. Those, who Dr. Bill sent, all came in wondering what the medicinal value of strawberry jam was, and had to be worked into our already full schedule.

One of the banes of medical practice was doing medical records at the hospital. In those days there were paper charts. When a patient was discharged, the doctor had to write up a discharge summary, make sure the chart had all the required signatures, and that it was complete and ship shape. This all had to be done within 2 weeks of the patient's departure, or the doctor would go on "the black list." That was the list that prevented them from admitting their patients to the hospital until their records were completed. No one wanted to end up on the black list since it would cause a serious issue with providing care for your patients. The one exception was medical service. Even if you were on the black list you still had to be on medical service. When you were on medical service, you had to take any and all patients who needed to be admitted but didn't have a regular doctor (likely because they also had no payment source). Those you still had to admit.

When one was on medical service, the challenge was always to find the last doctor who had touched that person for any reason. It was like he was "it." If you could find another doctor who had treated him before you, you might somehow convince the ER to call him for the admission. "That patient was obviously Dr. So and So's because he saw him last." The patient would be questioned. "Did Dr. So and So send you a letter dismissing you from his practice?" The answer was usually "No, he just wouldn't see me anymore because a) I didn't pay his bills, b) I never followed any of his instructions on taking medicines, c) I never kept my appointments, d) I went back to getting drunk or taking drugs and never saw him again or e) all of the above." "No? Then this is obviously Dr. So and So's patient." Unfortunately, when Dr. So and So was called, he might merely say, "He's not my patient. He was noncompliant, and I'm not seeing him," and hang up the phone. Then the doctor on medical service was responsible, no matter how undesirable the patient might be.

Now it was Dr. Bill who found a way around this arbitrary time of 2 weeks to get your records done or you're on the blacklist rule. He figured, if no one could <u>find</u> his charts, he couldn't be blacklisted and he was safe. So he deposited his incomplete charts in various draws, nooks and crannies all around the hospital. In order to suspend him, they had to find the charts. Once they found them, he would complete those that were found, and would never use that hiding place again. It was like a giant Easter egg hunt for the medical record staff every month. You had to hand it to him; the man was a master at this.

Now the way Al Capone had Eliot Ness, and Batman had the Joker, Dr. Bill had Dr. T. This Dr. T was the Sherlock Holmes of medical records. His mission was to catch Dr. Bill in the act of hiding his records and bust him. It was the proverbial cat and mouse game played out.

Dr. T was a family doc, who somehow came to be in charge of making sure the medical records were up to date and up to snuff, and therefore was not the most loved of physicians by his colleagues. He seemed to be more interested in other things than he was in practicing medicine, like how to make everybody else's life miserable. But catching Dr. Bill became his life's dream and obsession. If he could, Dr. T would have challenged Dr. Bill to a duel with pistols at 20 paces right in front of the hospital's main entrance, but it would have been unlikely that Dr. Bill would have taken him up on it, or would have shown up, even if he said he would. This rivalry just went to show how little commonality there is between someone who loves being a rule breaker out on the ocean fishing and someone who loves being a rule enforcer fishing through hospital records indoors. They were almost natural enemies from the start.

Drs. Y and Z were the highest earning family physicians in the area, with the biggest practices. Dr. Y and Z practiced together at one time, and developed a unique practice style. They used 6 exam rooms each and 2 nurses each. Each nurse would cover 3 rooms. Nurse #1 would bring patients into rooms 1, 2 and 3, take a brief history on each, and write it on the chart (for example sore throat or headache). Then she would accompany the doctor into the first 3 rooms. The doctor would do a problem specific exam, and while doing so, would dictate a prescription, which the nurse would write out. The doctor would sign it, the nurse would give it to the patient, and the visit was over. He'd make a brief note with the diagnosis ("pharyngitis") and treatment

("PenVK") and move on to the next room. While he was seeing the patients in the first 3 rooms, nurse #2 was cleaning rooms 4, 5 and 6 post visit, and then rooming the next 3 patients in her 3 rooms. They'd schedule one patient every 5 minutes for 5-6 hours. Their rule was one problem per visit. When I said I spent 15-20 minutes per patient for acute visits, and 30-45 minutes on other visits, I was told I was spending too much time with them. They said the patients wanted to get in and get out, and not be romanced by the doctor.

These visits must have been like magic tricks. While you were watching the doctor, he would vanish, and magically appear in the next room. Nowadays they do the same trick using computers. Symptom, *click*. Exam, *click*. Diagnosis, *click*. Treatment, *click*. ("You can pick up your prescription at your pharmacy.") Door open and closed. So in actuality, Drs. Y and Z were just ahead of their time—pioneers in the field of no nonsense, and no conversation, office visits. Back then they called it efficiency; today they call it cost control and electronic medical records.

I should probably tell you about their medical records system. The patients' medical records were index cards, with the name in the top left or right corner. Each visit was one line: date, complaint, diagnosis and treatment. Lest you think that this was unusual, this system was the preferred one in use in almost all of the rural practices at that time. And if you think that the medical records were inadequate by today's standards, understand that these physicians lived with their patients. They knew the family history, past history, and social history. In fact the whole town usually knew this information. Many a story would begin with "when the Hansons all got the chicken pox," or "right after Harold got divorced from Helen," or "just after Mabel had her appendix out," or "if Mike would just stop drinking...." Illnesses were swapped like baseball cards at town get-togethers. "Oh, yeah, diabetes definitely runs in that family" or "Don't count on him being around long. They all die of heart attacks by the time they're 50" or "They've been married 3 years already. I wonder why they haven't had any children" were commonly overheard conversations.

Then there was the medical illness one-upmanship. "You think that's a rash? Let me show you what I've got. Now *this is a rash!*" "You think getting attacked by a wolverine is painful? Well, then you've never gotten your foot caught in a bear trap." "Oh, yeah, well when I was in the hospital they took out my appendix without anesthesia." "You think that's a scar. Look at what they gave me." Privacy for medical issues and conditions wasn't even a thought.

Drs. Y and Z had a falling out years before I got to town. It was about whose patient was whose. "That patient always sees me. How come she's in your schedule?" and "I can't help it if she prefers to see me, and asks to see me. I'm not going to tell her no" was how the battle would start; first with small volleys, then with cannon and heavy artillery.

After they split, the same arguments would be heard in the hospital hallways, when one found out the other had admitted the other's patient. I figured that what they needed to do is to have their patients branded, like the cows out west. And patients would need to know that they were not allowed to drift around between doctors and/or health care facilities. "Check the brand. Did they have the Rockin' R or the Bar W brand on them?" All parties would also have to know that patient rustling was a hanging offense. If they were found in another doctor's exam room, the doctor could pay the ultimate price for rustling. What was really baffling was that each of these physicians had more patients than either of them could handle alone. You'd think they'd be thankful for the break once in a while.

Another doctor in town was Dr. B. He was a general surgeon. The product of a Jewish father and an Irish Roman Catholic mother, he was told he could choose his religion when he became of age. Consequently, he chose none of the above. However, he did inherit his father's Jewish sense of humor, and his mother's Irish gift of blarney. He was therefore a natural born entertainer. He would be the MC at any event, and would tell jokes and introduce the other acts. He could have been another Billy Crystal if he hadn't chosen medicine.

He would regale all with his Mo and Abie jokes. The jokes were quite good. I remember some of them even today:

> Mo and Abie were arguing about whether there was life after death, and they finally agreed that, if one of them died, he would come back to the other one, if he could, and tell the remaining one what life was like after death. As it happened, Mo died first. Every day Abie would wait to hear from Mo, but he didn't come back. Then one day, one year after Mo died, Abie hears his name called one night. "Abie, Abie." "Who's there?" "Abie. It's me, Mo." "Mo, you've come back. Tell me, what's it like?" "Abie, let me tell you what it's like. The sky is always blue, and you can see for miles." "Mo, what about the food? Is the food good there?" "The food, they just keep bringing it. More food than you can possibly eat." "Mo, tell me, are there women?" "Women! There are more than I can keep up with. A new one every day." "So, Mo, you're telling me you're in heaven?" "Heaven? No. I'm reincarnated as a bull on a ranch in Montana."
>
> Another joke was about 2 priests who died the same day in an auto accident, and went up to St. Peter. When they met him, St. Peter told them that with all the natural disasters around the world, he was backed up checking people in, and they would have to go back to earth for a few days, till he got caught up with the back log. He told them they could go back to earth and be anything they wanted to be. The first priest knew exactly what he wanted. He said he wanted to be an eagle. He wanted to be able to soar over the mountains of the earth. "Done," said St. Peter, and the first priest vanished. The other priest wasn't so sure. He wanted some clarification. He said, "Now we're in right? No matter what we do now, it won't affect our coming back." St. Peter assured him that his place was safe in heaven, no matter what happened on earth over the next few days. "In that case," the priest said, "I want to be a stud." "Done," said St. Peter, and the second one vanished. After a few days, St. Peter called an angel to pick up the 2 priests, and bring them back. "The first one is an eagle in

northern Idaho. He'll be easy to find soaring around. The other will be more difficult. He's embedded in a snow tire in Vermont."

Dr. B had to have coronary artery bypass surgery when he was about 50 yrs. old, for which he felt fortunate, because during the surgery, they discovered he had a small esophageal cancer, which they removed and treated. Unfortunately this was a very aggressive form of cancer, and it came back, causing him to go through round after round of excruciating treatments. Once he was talking to me in the doctor's lounge about his attitude toward what seemed to be futile medical treatments and procedures. He quoted Dylan Thomas, saying that he would "not go gently into that good night but would rage against the dying light." I thought about this conversation quite a bit, wondering why he would continue seemingly useless treatments which just prolonged his suffering. The ethical arguments were debated by all the physicians about just ending it. Some felt that it was only God's prerogative to end a life. Other's felt they should be able to choose for themselves how, when and where they want to die. No one really knows what one would do or want to do if put in that same situation, but it is hard to imagine that death would be the answer to any problem related to suffering.

I do know people who went through the uncomfortable and perhaps useless treatments, not because they didn't want to die, but rather to stay around for those they love, and from whom they did not want to be separated.

Before he died, Dr. B converted to Roman Catholicism, received the sacraments and died in the good graces of the church. Some thought he did this because he wanted to make sure he would not be the one, who ended up being a bull in Montana.

Dr. S was the other general surgeon in town. He was from S. Korea, and was the only surgeon on staff who was not divorced or having an affair. He was what I had always imagined a surgeon was like. When called, even at 2 or 3 AM, he would always show up with a suit and tie on, while I was doing good to show up with a scrub suit on (generally what I slept in). When Dr. S came in, it was like he was just waiting at home to be called, just like the scenes one sees of the doctors in the movies or on TV. A made for TV moment.

Dr. S was always a gentleman and a great colleague. He always trusted his colleague's judgment and diagnosis. He never made them feel like they were idiots because they didn't know what the "cornrow sign" was, like others were apt to do. He would teach as well as consult. And he was just about unflappable. He could be presented the most bizarre case anyone had ever seen, and he would just nod and say, "We see this sometimes," even when everyone knew dang well he'd never seen anything close to this. He would operate on people that other surgeons would walk away from as hopeless. He would sometimes be up to his knees in blood, and pull the patient back from the jaws of death. And after doing so would just act like everything went according to plan, with a "We see this sometimes."

Dr. F was the typical absent minded professor. He was the only person any doctor had ever known who could forget that he had to take call on a particular night or weekend. One time when he was supposed to take call for a weekend, he called up his coverage group from Bermuda asking if someone could take the calls for him, because he was out of the country. He would promise to take any future date they chose in exchange, but, after agreeing to a date, he would promptly forget about it. Even though they may have hated him for being on the pink sands of Bermuda, while they were in the cold frozen tundra of another winter, they would agree to cover him. The problem was he was very likeable, so no one could ever get really mad at him for long even after he ruined everyone else's plans.

Perhaps the worst forgetting episode Dr. F had was when he forgot he was married, and started to live with another woman. When he was reminded that he had a previous obligation, he thought it would be just fine to have both his women live with him, together, in the same house, and no, he wasn't Mormon or Muslim, where such arrangements are perhaps tolerated. He couldn't understand why that just wouldn't work for all the other parties involved. (The party of the first part was not going to put up with the party of the third part, even if she was pregnant, and eventually didn't put up with the party of the second part either.) While he was putting everybody through this idiocy, his father came to town, and wanted to talk to me. Not being sure if his father thought that I had put him up to this, or had influenced him in some way to do this, I was naturally nervous about the meeting. When I met with him, the father shook my hand, sat down, and told me his son saw me as one of his good friends. Then he said, "What the hell is the matter with him? Do you have any idea? Has he lost his mind?" His father was devastated. He had raised his son to be a devout Quaker. He himself was on the board of directors of a Quaker college, and his son on the board of a Quaker day school. He was raised to know better. "We don't act like this. The man's been bewitched."

Dr. F's father knew that he could not live life for his son, nor could he make decisions for him, but by Jove, didn't he raise him to be better than this? Men do strange and incomprehensible things in the name of love. Dr. F was a father as well. When this occurred, his children were aged 10 and 11, old enough to understand what was going on. They couldn't understand why their daddy wanted them to have 2 mommies, and why this other woman was going to be giving them a new brother or sister. Dr. F's father wondered how they were going to react to this and what would happen after a divorce. Surely Dr. F wouldn't get custody of the children. Would his wife then move to some far-away place to escape from Dr. F and the shame he brought to his family? Would he to be able to continue to see his grandchildren? These thoughts weighed heavily on his mind.

The marriage finally ended when the party of the first part divorced the party of the second part for being an incorrigible polygamist and idiot. After which Dr. F left town with his new partner and without his children.

I should let you know that Dr. F's ex-wife had a happy ending though. She got remarried to her attorney, became the town selectman and by all accounts lived happily ever after.

Dr. F's partner, Dr. D, didn't have quite as happy of an ending. When Dr. F left town, Dr. D decided he couldn't deal with the work schedule by himself, left his medical practice altogether and went to work for an insurance company; thus, leaving a very big hole in the availability of physicians for our call schedule, which meant a lot more work for those of us family doctors who remained.

It was more than just a hole in the work schedule though to us. Dr. D was about the only doctor anyone knew who could put up with, and get along with, Dr. F's antics on a daily basis. In fact he could put up with anyone's antics. He was unflappable as well as affable. He was quick to laugh and joke, and always made the best of really bad situations. Dr. D had been in the Coast Guard before going to medical school, and would talk of those "great times when he was out in a storm in the North Atlantic. The ice cold wind would whip through the ship. The cold seemed to penetrate your very bones. The icy waves would break over the bow and wash over the deck, and the spray of the sea water would hit your face and feel like needles." He would make off the cuff comments, like "Yeah, once I was washed overboard and almost drowned," and then laugh an endearing laugh. "Yeah, compared to that, this is a night at the Ritz Carleton." He never complained. Whatever he was doing was better than being out in the North Atlantic taking on water in a storm. His absence in our group's call schedule was deeply felt.

Across town, Dr. L was a family doc who started a clinic with Dr. M. They were the first physicians in the area who actually worked together in the same office. When they first came to town in the 1950's, they were the new hot shots, who had just finished their training together. They were the first ones to introduce IV fluid treatments to the hospital. They even made their own solutions. Dr. L was crusty and opinionated, and would go toe to toe with anyone. When Dr. L was in a teaching hospital one time after having a heart attack, he knew exactly what kind of treatment he wanted and needed. It was said that a young intern, who was taking care of him, felt he was the one in charge of Dr. L's care, and didn't want to give Dr. L what he was asking for. That was when Dr. L asked the intern to get closer to him so he could tell him something confidentially. When the intern bent over to listen, Dr. L grabbed him by the throat, and told him he would choke the #&*% life out of him, if he didn't get the treatment he felt he needed. As the intern passed out, he agreed to his patient's terms. This was the beginning of patients being involved in their treatment decisions. That's just another example of being ahead of the time.

Dr. M took up motorcycle riding for the adventure of it, but also to be able to be alone when he wanted to. He would arrive at the hospital on his motorcycle, park in a no parking zone and walk into the hospital, and dared any security person to give him a ticket. One guard took him up on his dare, wrote a ticket out, and left it on the motorcycle. The next day Dr. M took the ticket up to the hospital administrator, told him there are no parking areas specifically for motorcycles, and until there were he would "park any $%#% place he pleased." He then ripped the ticket up, threw it on the administrator's desk and walked out. Later that week the guard, who wrote the ticket, was brought in to the administrator of the hospital and told to leave Dr. M and his motorcycle alone if he valued his job and a certain set of body parts. Dr. M received no more tickets.

Dr. E, a pathologist, was always in the doctor's lounge pushing a new way to avoid death and constipation. His latest solution to these great scourges of mankind was bran. Bran muffins, bran flakes, bran bread, bran in yogurt, bran on ice cream and bran in mashed potatoes. One day to drive home his point, he brought in some bran muffins that he made at home for everyone to taste. Now I always liked Dr. E, so as to not make him feel bad, I tried one of his muffins. "These muffins taste like sawdust," I told him. "Small price to pay for all the benefits," he replied.

Dr. P was a small town boy who did well for himself. He was locally born and bred. He went to the local schools and returned to his home town to practice. His whole family was very proud of him. Unfortunately his family was very large and now all figured they had a doctor on retainer. They called at all hours to "ask his opinion" about some medical issue or just dropped into his office to get checked out. That was all well and good, but they also didn't feel they should have to pay him anything because, after all, they were family.

Now while Dr. P was very unconcerned with this situation, his wife felt that he was being taken advantage of. And she made no bones about venting her anger at this, particularly at family gatherings. She was not above calling them a "bunch of freeloaders and leeches" very loudly and very clearly so everyone could hear. But she could not insult them enough to make them find another doctor to go to. However, she did get her way when she convinced Dr. P to specialize, which in fact he did. After he did, not one of his family members would come to see him or want it to become known by anyone that they were seeing Dr. P. You see he specialized in sexually transmitted diseases.

The most interesting doctors of all those in town were perhaps those in the Radiology Department. There were 3 Irish docs there who had immigrated together from Ireland—Murphy, Fitzgerald and O'Toole. The rumor was that they were members of the Irish Republican Army back in their home country. They were very gregarious and always ready to have a beer and a laugh with you.

Murphy married an American woman, and was losing some of his fire for fighting and dying for a free Ireland. Fitzgerald brought his wife to the U.S. from Ireland. She was happy to be in a country where her husband was not at war with anyone, and encouraged him to leave well enough alone. "You've no relations there anymore. It's not personal anymore. Just be happy here," she would tell him. But O'Toole was still in the trenches. He never got married, and made sure he was always able to answer the call. O'Toole was the most outspoken about his beliefs. "If the Queen were here right now, I'd spit in her eye, and wouldn't think twice about it," he would say. Just because they were in the former colonies that had won their independence from Britain, didn't mean that they should stop trying to win Irish independence. They weren't happy that almost all of Ireland was free. Unless Northern Ireland was free of British rule, none of Ireland was free, according to their way of thinking. He bought a goodly piece of land and built a house that had more security than the White House. Packages would leave his house with warnings like "Handle with extreme care" and "Do not drop" written on them. The UPS drivers would wonder what exactly could be in them. When they would ask Dr. O'Toole what he was sending to Ireland, he would just say, "Some very delicate equipment," and leave it at that.

A strange thing happened one night that had the whole town talking. About 3 AM there was a tremendous explosion at Dr. O'Toole's house. It seemed a few men were trying to breach his fence, hit a trip wire, and got blown to smithereens. When investigated, it was noted that they were not from the area, and had no identification on them. The state police were very interested in the reason Dr. O'Toole had so much C-4 plastic explosives around his house. He said "it was just a hobby" of his and left it at that. But a couple of days later, he told his partners in radiology, that "they'd found him" and he was going to be leaving. And then he simply vanished. His house was up for sale a long time before some investor bought it and converted it into a guns, ammo and army surplus store. It was thought an appropriate tribute to Dr. O'Toole.

The Rest

Each doctor had his own quirks and interests. The pathologist, who loved Gilbert and Sullivan, would star in local productions. An internist, who really wanted to be a farmer, grew monster pumpkins, which he would enter in the town fair every year, and sometimes win. There were some docs, who came down from Canada to escape the onerous socialized health care system up there. There was the doc who always slept through the medical staff meetings, the one who brought up "parliamentary points of procedure," which kept the meetings going on forever, the doc who always showed up late and left early and of course those who carried their own self-importance like they were afraid of breaking it.

The ER

When I first started practicing, the ER at the hospital had hired one ER doc, a local boy who had done good and just finished school. When he got a patient who had anything more complicated than a cold, he liked to have company. He'd call you in, anytime day or night, to "manage ***your*** patient," with the emphasis on "your." In those days all the doctors would admit and manage their own patients in the hospital. There was no strictly hospital based practice, like today.

Now I don't mean to be hard on this ER doc. When you're in the ER everyone knows all your mistakes. And when you were born, raised and live in a town like Bainbridge, everyone in town also knows. You can forever be remembered and identified by one mistake, and it will be passed on down to the 4th generation. The story will start, "Remember when Harry went to the ER and DP was on duty?" When that begins, you have gotten yourself a reputation, which you may have to leave town in order to get rid of.

When he was off they hired some retired family docs, who were great. They'd take care of the patients, and if they needed to be admitted, would even write some holding orders, so you didn't have to stop whatever it was you were doing, and rush right in to see them. They came from out of town, were a whole lot more experienced and didn't have home town issues.

The Pediatricians

Although the pediatricians were by and large a very easy going lot, and easy to work with, they were detested by some of the other docs. This wasn't due to their medical care, but rather from artificially contrived economics of the situation. It started when the first pediatricians, who were in private practice, were unable to make a living because of all the family docs already in the area. The hospital felt it was important to have 'pediatricians.' So in order to keep a pediatrician presence in the hospital, the hospital board decided to hire the current pediatrician, as well as hire another 2 for coverage, and subsidize them. This was the first known occurrence of a doc being "bought" by the hospital. There was talk of the hospital owning a "stable of physicians," and driving private practice out of business, which is exactly what happened over the next 40 years. Private and independent physician offices became almost non-existent.

Up until this time most docs went to an area set up their practices, and stayed there their whole lives. Primary care doctors, or generalists, were the main caregivers for whole families, with a gradual shift toward more specialists coming in to cherry pick certain patients needing more advanced care in a certain area. However, with this hospital-owned practice model, we would have docs, who came into town, practiced for 2-3 years, and then left for somewhere else. I couldn't imagine starting a practice all over again. The set up costs, the credentialing, and just the moving were daunting to me. Then I found out the reason behind the moves. These docs were offered a large "signing bonus," and a guarantee of a minimum income by the hospital to practice in the area for at least 2 or 3 years, about the time it takes for a practice to become profitable (thinking, of course, that once they established a practice for 2 or 3 years, they'd stay in town). But after their time stipulation was up, they'd go to another place, and get another signing bonus, and would do this over and over.

I never thought I would know so much about the lives of my colleagues. But small towns have a culture where secrets are meant to be found out. All the flaws a person has are on display for everyone to see. It was a way of keeping everyone humble. One couldn't think of themselves as better than someone else when everyone else knew better, and that's the way it was going to stay, because that's the way everyone liked it. I was sure that I, or my own family, would come up with some incident or two that would be the talk of the town at some point, so I wouldn't be surprised when it occurred—only embarrassed. It was just the nature of mankind. Some would call it the sinful nature that makes men race toward their own destructions and unhappiness, all the while thinking they are pursuing happiness, and all the while making poor choices and bad decisions. The thing that always amazes me is the fact that those decisions are deliberate and willful. They are not errors or mistakes. We walk in with our eyes wide open.

The Nurses

The nurse, who cared for your patients in the hospital, could be your best friend or your worst enemy. The places they could critically affect your life as a doctor, were in the ICU and Maternity. When I first started, the ICU was basically 6 beds in the same room with 2 nurses. The beds weren't even all monitored at that time. The nurse was the first to alert you that there may be trouble brewing, and would suggest some action be taken to head any problem off at the pass. They were inevitably right. Maternity was another area where the nursing care could make or break you. They were the ones monitoring a laboring patient, would alert you if things weren't progressing as expected, and let you know when you needed to come in for the delivery. One particular nurse was extremely anxious, always expected trouble and, unfortunately, always worked at night. She would call you every 10 minutes until, finally convinced you'd get more sleep at the hospital than at home, you'd go in.

The winters were usually brutally cold and snowy with below zero temperatures and snow depth measured in feet. Having to shovel out the car and scrapping off the windows was getting old for me. The worst was having to go out in the middle of the night to deliver a baby that wasn't going to wait. One time I was called by the OB nurse, notifying me that my patient had checked in, and was in early labor. The next thing I knew, I had a State Trooper outside my home ringing the bell and knocking on the door loudly. As I made my way to the door, I could see the cruiser's lights flashing. I couldn't imagine what was going on. When I got the door opened, the cop told me the hospital was trying to get in touch with me, and I had to get in there to deliver a baby. I discovered that after I had last spoken to the nurse, I had fallen back to sleep with the phone in my hand.

Another night I went to bed with the snow again falling. I got a call from the OB nurse telling me I needed to come in. I asked the nurse I was speaking to if it was still snowing. "What do I look like? The weather lady?" was her response. "Just get in here." Lesson: If you want any comfort or consolation, don't expect to get it from an OB nurse attending to a woman in active labor.

CHAPTER 7

The Office

After hospital rounds I went to the office. Since I was still paying off the loans, which I took out to furnish the exam rooms, the office was sparsely decorated. The waiting room had dark blue cushioned chairs and wood paneling on the wall. The carpeting was wearing out at the doorway as well as where folks stood at the receptionist's counter. One thing I did provide my patients with was magazines to read that were all up to date. No copies from 1969. Along with the required *This Old House, Farm and Garden, American Rifleman, Field and Stream, Birds and Blooms, Life, Saturday Evening Post and Yankee,* I added an eclectic mix of my interests, *American Patriot, The Christian Family, Touchstone* and *The New Oxford Review* to name a few. I figured that if they're going to be waiting, they may as well have something worthwhile to look at and maybe get educated.

The patients in my office were greeted by Madeline, the receptionist. Madeline was a local girl, born and bred in town. If you went back far enough, she was related to almost everyone. Because of her multitude of relations, for a short period of time, she seemed to become a professional mourner and funeral attender. Prior to that, she was the professional wedding and baptism attender. We made her the official ambassador for the office for all these occasions.

Madeline was one of those people who could not say no to anyone, including those who were seeking an appointment with the doctor. She would say, "Why don't you come in about 5 PM and we'll work you in." So around 5 o'clock when we thought we were winding down for the day, we would find an extra 10-12 patients waiting to be "worked in."

One thing was for certain, I never lacked for patients while Madeleine worked for us. But not lacking for patients did not translate necessarily into not lacking for paying patients. The number of patients seen was not the same as the number of patients who paid for services. Our collection percentage was below 80%, which was fine for keeping the business solvent, but not enough to allow me to provide for upgrading or any increases in salaries. But Madeline was certainly doing her part to keep the patients flowing into the office.

Our nurse, Wendy, filled the roll of nurse and practice manager. She was the one who kept things flowing—ordered supplies, screened incoming phone calls, roomed patients and assisted with procedures. She was extremely efficient, and I was fortunate to have her. Wendy was willing to work long hours and stay late, a very rare find. I always brought Wendy in for the most unpleasant procedures, like draining an abscess, the smell of which would gag a maggot, or fishing out a tampon that was lost for a month in some woman's nether regions. Usually after these procedures, the room would be unusable, and would have to be aired out. As patients would pass the room, we would hear comments like "Good God, what's that smell?" or "What did somebody die in there?" or "Whoa, you've got to get that body buried." Or, best of all, "Smells like low tide."

Wendy was not from this town, so she did not know all the background and family connections, like Madeline did, but she was a fast learner. She knew exactly which patients were going to need extra time—those who'd want or need to talk about the events in their lives, their political persuasions or their religious beliefs. She knew which ones would be coming in with a laundry list of symptoms, numbering anywhere from 6 to 12. And she knew which would be quick because they had to get to back to work, or get back home to meet the school bus. She was a wizard at keeping patients flowing through the office, in the least amount of time possible, given the circumstances.

The search for good help, those knowledgeable, efficient and dedicated, was not an easy one. In the hiring process, one girl, who was hired to be a receptionist, didn't work out because she was giving out medical advice over the phone, without asking me or Wendy. They would be considered home remedies or the "grandma always used to..." type of advice. Some remedies were very suspect. ("Just take 3 teaspoons of a mixture of honey, lemon and vinegar and that strep throat should clear right up." Or "Just rub some bacon grease on that burn." Or "One ounce of apple cider vinegar 4 times a day should fix that upset stomach right up." Or "Take a candle, light it and drip the wax in your ear and that will take care of that earache." Or "Put a little kerosene on that poison ivy rash.") Another newly hired receptionist just disappeared from her post, and was found in the closet crying her eyes out, saying she couldn't take the pressure. Most of the women, who applied for the job, thought being a receptionist meant answering the phone every once in a while (not every minute as was the reality) and reading a book or eating bonbons in their free time. They were in shock when they discovered there was no free time.

The Drug Reps

At this time the drug reps were welcomed. Some became like part of the family, stopping in to drop off donuts or bring lunch, and ask if we needed any samples for our patients who couldn't afford their prescriptions. Occasionally they would have a dinner with a guest speaker, who would tell us the latest and greatest about their newest product. At that time we were allowed to bring wives or family, if they wanted to be bored by the speaker. After a couple of these, my wife had had it, so I brought my son. He liked to hang around with the "big boys," and he would listen intently to the speaker, who was usually from India, and spoke English with an accent. I let him come until he, himself, began talking with an Indian accent. I just didn't need to be answering this question: "Why does your son speak with an accent? Did you adopt him from India?"

The Medical Students

During my time in practice, the University School of Medicine was embarking on a program whereby all third year students would spend a month with a practicing family physician. I expressed an interest in being a mentor for these students and, after being vetted, was selected as a community practice site. This was not a particularly popular clerkship with all the students, especially with those who already decided you couldn't pay them enough to be family doctors. Plus in order to get to my practice they had to drive at least 45-60 minutes 4 days/week. To cut down on their driving time, we offered to put them up in a spare bedroom, but even then, not everyone was overjoyed to come out.

I would have them perform some minor procedures in the office and interview patients, but that was not the main skill I wanted them to acquire. I would tell all the med students that came: "You can learn how to take care of a heart attack from the cardiologist, how to take care of hard to manage diabetes from the endocrinologist, how to take care of MS from the neurologist, but I'm here to teach you how to take care of people. What you are seeing in your office is not hypertension, high cholesterol, diabetes or sore throats. You are seeing Mrs. Jones with hypertension, Mr. Smith with diabetes and Johnny Jones with a sore throat. You have to know them as people, who they are, what they believe in, what they value, and who they are connected to and supported by. They have to know that you care about them as people. They won't care what you know, unless they first know you care. Once you know them, and care about them, then you can start to take care of their medical problems. Your patients will teach you much about life and death, by just giving you the privilege of letting you be with them during some of their hardest times and helping them through it." Needless to say, their interviewing and history taking skills needed to be a little different from what they learned in med school.

The first student assigned to me was Steve, a guy from California who had already decided he would NOT be going into family practice. However, he was single, and took us up on our offer to stay at our house during his clerkship. Since he stayed with us, he saw family practice first hand—all of it. When called out at night, he came with me. When we worked late, he worked late. He played ping pong with my kids, ate dinner with us, and occasionally would watch TV with us.

One night we were called out for a delivery. I had Steve help with the delivery of the baby, and cut the cord. That was a night I'll never forget, even if he has long forgotten it. He came home so excited, he could barely contain himself. He kept saying what a wonderful experience he had just had, and just could not stop talking about it. Needless to say, there was no sleep to be gotten that night. When he graduated, he decided to go into family practice, and is still practicing in Washington.

He was my only success story, if one measures success by who went on to be family doctors. All the others remained committed to their specialties. But I would hope they are all better physicians because of the time they spent with me.

Barbara

Barbara was a 50 year old lady, who I had taken care of for many years. Over the many years that I cared for her, I just could not impact or lessen her self-destructive behavior patterns. She was 300 lbs., a diabetic on insulin, and yet drank liters of Coke per day, ate donuts by the dozens, and cookies as part of her normal diet. I was convinced she actually had a physical addiction to donuts— a donutaholic, if you will. If she started a box of a dozen donuts, she couldn't stop eating them until they were all gone. She was also having breathing trouble because of her habit of smoking 2 packs of cigarettes a day, yet she wouldn't, or couldn't, stop. She was afraid of losing her legs because she had diabetes, and yet would allow them to swell to 3 times normal size, and not take care of her skin.

When I tried to talk to her about these things, she'd give me a smile, like someone who got caught with their hand in the cookie jar. Her daughter would come with her to her appointments, and she, along with me, would try to come up with some plan to help her mother, but Barbara would thwart each and every one of them.

After being frustrated with this situation over many years, I finally said, "Look, maybe it's time for you to find a new doctor. Obviously I haven't helped you very much. I can't seem to help you stop smoking, or to modify your eating in order to keep you healthy. Maybe you should try to find a different doctor, who can do a better job to get you motivated to live a healthier lifestyle."

Barbara just looked at me incredulously and said, "What are you crazy? Who else do you think is going to put up with me? I'm not an easy patient, you know."

After years of this, she finally ended up in a nursing home. When she got there, she thought she was at a spa with servants. She wanted everything, and I mean everything, done for her. It took a monumental effort to get her out of the bed and into a wheelchair every day. She wouldn't walk, because it was too difficult. She wouldn't eat what she was supposed to, because she didn't like it. Her boyfriend who came to visit her was like her drug dealer bringing in contraband foods from home. Every so often, the nursing staff would conduct a raid in her room, and find candy bars hidden amongst her things, scattered all around the room. But that never stopped her supplier from getting her another shipment. It became a game to see if she could find a place where the nurses couldn't find them.

But the one thing she wanted to do, more than anything, was to smoke. But when a non-smoking policy was instituted in the facility, she could only smoke when someone on the nursing staff could find the time to wheel her outside in her oversized wheelchair. This was not done as frequently as she demanded, and was usually undertaken by a staff member who also wanted to smoke. It was at this point I came up with a plan to modify her behavior.

The solution: she and the nursing staff were told that the only way she could smoke was if she *walked* outside, and it had to be under her own power. No wheelchairs. It was weeks later that I received the following fax.

Since Barbara started smoking the following observations have been noted:

1. *ambulation has increased from 2 ft. to 150 ft. to reach the smoking area*
2. *swelling in her legs has decreased from severe (4+) to minimal (1+)*
3. *her weight has gone down from 306 lbs. to 293 lbs.*
4. *the wounds on her legs have almost completely healed*
5. *she is tolerating being off oxygen for longer periods of time*
6. *her diabetes is well controlled*

Would you like us to encourage smoking to improve others as well?? ☺

(Signed) Jan Harper

Jan was a nurse who had as much of an addiction to smoking as Barbara. Every time I went to visit Barbara at the nursing home, I spent just as much time talking to Jan about her quitting smoking. It was costing her a small fortune, and she could ill afford the expense. Because of that expense, she began taking trips to the Native American (formerly Indian) Casino, where she could buy cigarettes by the case for less, and avoid paying taxes at the same time. Now as the population grew, the need for services grew. As the need for services grew, the need for tax money increased. So the state decided to collect some of the sales taxes on out of state purchases or purchases at tax free casinos. The tax rule was written so that even if you paid for something tax free in another state, like New Hampshire, one was still liable to pay the State of Connecticut the sales tax. The citizens were told they were required to report these sales and pay the taxes. So the state would stake out the casinos and watch for cars coming out of the casinos and take down the plate numbers.

One day Jan got a notice from the State IRS that told her she owed $10,000 to the state for sales taxes she had not been paying including penalties and interest. It seems that after getting her license plate number, connecting it to her name, they then ran her credit cards and found purchases at the Casino. They then extrapolated this number for the past 5 years and came up with her tax bill. She tried to fight the tax, but the state had way more resources and tax attorneys than she did. So she began working overtime to pay for her habit and her taxes. One of her co-workers suggested that she move out of the country, but that seemed a little drastic to Jan. She was not opposed to finding someone rich to marry, but that didn't seem to be happening. The closest she got was when one of the old men, who resided in the nursing home, propositioned her, but he was on state assistance. As luck would have it, Jan struck a friendship with one of the state IRS agents who were investigating her. They started dating and finally got married. She stopped smoking, and moved to Tennessee, where there is no state income tax, and lived happily ever after by all accounts.

I Want to See Your Soul

Observing my elderly patients, I noticed that many seemed so frail, and while their physical capacities diminished, their minds stayed sharp and their interests remained keen. Some would make comments like "I don't even recognize that person I see in the mirror" or "I don't remember growing old. When did it happen?" One day I asked one of them, after they told me they looked old but didn't really feel old inside, "How old do you feel inside?" "About 20." It struck me at that time that what I was seeing was the person's body, but not their soul. The soul never ages, therefore never feels old or looks old. So I began asking my patients, who were 65 years of age or older, if they wouldn't mind bringing in a picture of themselves when they were between 18 and 25 years old. It could be a wedding picture, graduation picture, military picture or just a casual snapshot. When I was asked why, as I inevitably was, I would tell them, "I want to see your soul. Your soul is always young and beautiful. And I wanted everyone else to see you as young, as you are inside."

By doing this I got lots of pictures, and with each picture came a story about when the picture was taken, what they were doing, where they were and many events I never would have heard about otherwise. I received wedding pictures, high school graduation pictures, pictures in military uniforms taken during WWII, and professional and candid pictures. These pictures were opportunities to see these people in a new light and to understand them better. It helped me and others understand that everyone has an interesting story. And every story is important to hear because, to the person telling their story, it's the only one they have. And it's important to them.

Not everyone was happy with this. One day a woman was in the office, and noticed her mother's picture on our bulletin board, with her name and date. She looked at it, and then turned to the receptionist and said, "I don't even have this picture." She continued by saying something like "How dare he take my mother's picture!" and proceeded to take it off the board and put in into her pocketbook. When I noticed the gaping hole on the board with the missing picture, I asked if anyone knew what happened to it. (There actually was some deliberate vandalism to some of the pictures by others who didn't like, or had issues with, those pictured. Hard to believe but true.)

My receptionist told me what had happened. I then wrote to the patient's daughter, and told her if she had wanted the picture, all she had to do was ask. I would have been happy to give it to her, especially if she didn't have a copy of it. I would have even made some copies of it for her, if she would have liked. But she denied me the joy of giving her that picture by just taking it. The woman never answered that letter, and never came back to the office. Whether it was due to guilt, anger, hate, or shame I never found out.

CHAPTER 8

Coaching Little League

When my sons were about 7 years old and in the town Little League, their team was looking for a coach. My friend, Bob, agreed to coach my son's team, only if I would be the assistant coach. Now Bob was a professional coach, if only for the high school football team, and I was only a warm body to fill a slot. Unfortunately, we had a practice scheduled that Bob would not be able to make, and I was to fill in. In my delusion, I figured what could go wrong? Hit a few balls, let the kids catch, throw, and bat a little. It didn't take long for things to fall apart. The worst part was that there were parents there watching it all fall apart.

It began with a lazy fly ball to the outfielder. The kid in center field had it all the way, until it went past his glove, and hit him right between the eyes. The sound of the ball hitting his head seemed to echo throughout the field, and the spectators all gasped in unison. Luckily he was not knocked unconscious, but had a large egg sprouting on his forehead. Being a doctor, I called for the emergency kit, and for some ice. No ice was found, but in the emergency kit there was one of these chemical packs, that when you broke it, it became a cold pack. Breaking the cold pack, I applied it to his face. It was then that it was noticed by everyone that the chemicals from the cold pack were leaking out and into his eye, as he started screaming that his eye was burning. I think it was at that point that the kid's parents had had enough, and took him to the Emergency Room. I'm happy to report the kid was fine, and I was never asked to run a practice from that time on.

Team Doctor

I became the "team doctor" for Thornfield Hall, a residence for mentally and developmentally challenged girls, who, with very little effort on their parts, grew into old women - because of all the good medical and personal care they were receiving. I also became the doctor for the Jackson Center, a residential center for severely disabled young people, thus earning the title of the retarded doctor in town. Now the way I came to be asked to be the medical doctor for the Jackson Center was interesting. The patients had previously been taken care of by a pediatrician, who was about to retire, or at least retire from that position. It was a "thankless, difficult, demanding and low paying job," his words not mine. One day after coming to town, my wife and I went to the center, and asked them what they did, just to be familiar with the place. They took us for a tour, showed us the facility, and introduced us to some of the staff. When the time came to replace the medical director, they thought of me, because I was the only doctor who had ever shown any interest in the place.

It's amazing how things work out. During my residency I had virtually no experience, nor interest, in taking care of these sorts of patients, and yet now I was being handed a large group of them, and being told to take care of "the least of these."

I also became the physician for the Acme Cotton Mill, which made medical supplies, and for which I took over after its physician left the area. At this time there were many working mills in the area, although they would all eventually close up, and each had their own physician for their workers who became injured. Because of this I was asked to be the physician for Frito Lay, when they built a plant near Acme, and then Staples. Being a company physician was thought to be a plum job. Some paid a small stipend, and they referred you their workers who got injured at work. These were Workman's Comp cases, which generally required lots of paper work, for which you received very delayed payments. It also placed me in a position that made me uncomfortable. I was the company physician. The company's best interest was to have the patient either made better so they could get back to work as soon as possible, or declare him a malingerer – someone fit for work but just doesn't want to work. Anything that got him off Workman's Comp payments would do. Now came the conflict: the patient claimed he was still unable to work, but the company thought he was trying to milk the system and should be cleared for work. I guess I didn't side with the company enough, because I was eventually replaced at each company by a more compliant company physician.

At Acme I worked with the plant nurse, J.R., at least a couple of times a month to go over the safety issues at the plant. Her husband was a state policeman. Once I told her that on the way over to Acme I had just witnessed a car with teenage boys driving recklessly and terrorizing a group of nuns driving down the interstate. Her response was classic, "Where's a cop when you need one?" I eventually got the privilege of taking care of her whole family, including her parents and in-laws. I really liked JR and thought she was a good nurse, but shortly after I was let go by Acme, she was let go. Maybe they thought she was colluding with me on the patients we didn't agree on.

I also became a medical examiner and a police surgeon. The medical examiner at that time was called out for all deaths that were unattended by a physician, in order to pronounce them, determine the time of death and fill out a death certificate. You had to fill out a 4 page form for each pronouncement, for which you received a few dollars from the state. When you went to pronounce the person, you also had to call the chief medical examiner's office for them to determine whether they wanted to do an autopsy and get a number for the case. If there was a shooting or a bullet involved, they considered it a suspicious death (you think?) and would request the body be sent to them. Once I arrived at a home, and found a man in bed and quite dead. When I called the ME's office, I was told it wasn't suspicious, and I could release the body. As hard as I tried to convince them that the man may have been poisoned (I mean how would you know? Haven't they seen those murder mysteries?), they wouldn't change their mind. In the course of this, I would meet a lot of policemen, because they would have to stay with the body until I got there and released it. When the police called, they generally wanted you to get there as soon as possible, so their officer could get back to work. My argument, particularly during my working day, was that I couldn't just leave off taking care of the living in order to take care of the dead. I would generally get there in an hour or 2, but they were not happy with that. The actual policeman on duty there could care less. He was getting paid either way.

I also joined the Air National Guard, which gave me a little extra income, with the intent of putting in 20 years and retiring with a pension. That didn't happen. I had to get out after 4 years (the time required) or the Guard would have ruined my private practice. The clinic in the Guard was basically for airmen who were sick, or thought they were sick, and wanted to be released from duty, those who needed annual physicals or those who had some injury while on duty. The sergeants/medics ran that clinic like none I'd ever been in. At 12 noon they would go out into the waiting area and announce, "Lunch hour. Come back at 1300 hours." And everyone would leave, and form a new queue when they got back. At 1630 hours, they'd go out again, and say, "Clinic's closed." And everybody would go home. I've never had the pleasure of dealing with discretionary patients before or since.

The most remarkable thing that happened, while I was in the Guard, was the discovery that the Lt Col doctor in charge was not a doctor at all. He came from some country in SE Asia. He falsified all his documents, which I guess was easily done in that part of the world, if you bribed the right person. He had no license of any kind, and unbelievably also had a private practice in his town. Needless to say, when it was discovered, his playing doctor days were over. What this showed me was how important the work of the sergeants was. It was enough to even cover for an incompetent doctor and make him seem respectable.

Shortly after I came into town I was asked to become the medical advisor for the District Dept. of Health. It became a venue for me to speak to different groups about health issues. They would put on programs for various groups, and I would be invited to talk about whatever the topic was—high blood pressure, high cholesterol, heart attacks, strokes, diabetes or whatever they were interested in learning about.

I think I was invited to this position as a result of the local campaign to put fluoride in the water. The local pediatric dentist was advocating for the water to be fluorinated in order to reduce cavities in children. It was a long standing joke that upon high school graduation, the graduate got his diploma and a set of dentures. Whether this was because of lack of fluoride in the drinking water or just bad mouth care was debated. In any case the lines were drawn between the "progressives" and the "conservatives." This dentist called me, and asked if I would be willing to speak on the pro side, before the city commission, which was hearing the pro and con arguments of putting fluoride in the water. I think my remarks were the single most powerful reason for their decision to ***not*** put fluoride in the water. We had noted when we first came to town that the water in Bainbridge had an awful taste. You had to disguise it in some way, which was one reason the scotch and whiskey sales where booming. During my remarks, I flippantly said (never say anything flippantly in front of a gathering of town fathers and decision makers) that "adding fluoride would not detract from the great taste of the water, in so far as nothing could make it taste worse." The next day the only coverage in the newspaper on my testimony was about that comment. I guess the DDH thought anyone willing to say something that stupid was the person to be their medical advisor. Nowhere to go but up from here.

The second foray, that got my name in the newspaper, seemed like a reasonable request to me. At the time we were going to an Episcopal Church in Richmond, and my wife was teaching Sunday school. She mentioned to me that the boys never showed up during hockey season (which went from Sept.-May), because they had Sunday morning practices and games. I asked if some other time could be found for the boys to play/practice hockey, aside from Sunday morning, as that was the ONLY time they could get their religious instructions. They said that Sunday morning was the ONLY time they could get ice time.

Now I've heard all the arguments for kids participating in sports: it's healthy, it gives them exercise, keeps them out of trouble, gives them a preferable peer group, develops skills and may even get them a college scholarship. All of which I totally agree with. My only question is: "Does this have to take place on Sunday morning? Is there no other time?"

I contacted the Catholic priests, asking for support in reducing or eliminating Sunday morning activities for the kids programs, and was told, "They can go to church on Sat. afternoon, and they have their religious instructions on days other than Sunday. We don't have a problem with it." It was good to know that the priests were going to back us up on this. I guess if they thought that the kids were going to be taught heresy on Sunday, it's better that they not get to hear it at all. It's this kind of attitude that spawned the Protestant Reformation.

I was on the vestry (the committee to help run church business - yeah, I know, big mistake) at the time, and I composed a letter outlining that Sunday morning had been the traditional time to worship God and gather for fellowship and Bible teaching. Given this, I suggested that Sunday morning be kept free of children's activities. I also encouraged other churches to speak out against this Sunday morning activity trend, to discourage those planning such events, and (this was the lightning rod issue) for parents to not allow their children to participate in activities conducted on Sunday morning. Some other vestry members agreed, and we signed the letter, and sent it to the newspaper. The letter was gleefully published, as there is nothing newspapers like better than controversy.

Now one would expect that a politically liberal community, with "kind, compassionate and tolerant people," would react with a reasonable civil discourse. And, of course, one would be wrong. Instead we were regaled with letters and comments filled with vitriol, contempt and lectures on the true meaning of keeping, or rather not keeping, the Sabbath. Even members of our own congregation were dismissive at best. ("My child plays sports on Sunday morning, and I don't see anything wrong with it." "The Sabbath was made for man, not man for the Sabbath.")

Luckily our pastor weathered the storm I had created, and the Sunday activities, not only continued, but increased. It came to encompass, not only hockey, but also soccer, baseball and football in the coming years. The churches emptied on Sundays and the sporting venues filled. As the sports fields become the new cathedrals, which served hot dogs and beer, instead of bread and wine (although recently churches have skipped the bread and wine and now mostly just serve coffee and donuts), it is no wonder why the integrity of our young folks evaporated. One thing that athletes are not consistently exposed to is good sportsmanship and integrity of character—the only thing that matters now is winning. So it becomes acceptable to find subtle ways to cheat in order to gain an advantage over another team. The players no longer need to be a paragon of virtue and role models for our young people. Prison sentences, girlfriend and wife abuse is accepted if you're a great running back. Drug and alcohol use is frowned upon, but not enough to prevent a great wide receiver from playing and helping his team win a championship. Minor traffic offenses are totally overlooked. Only murder keeps you out of professional sports and sometimes not even then.

My first foray into the field of popular culture was a complete and utter failure. But did that discourage me? No. I was a glutton for punishment in that area.

D&D

Another time my name was in the papers was related to a game called Dungeons and Dragons. A game I had never heard of until that time. It was this event that got me involved in the culture wars. I became a proponent of Christian morals, and of the values that I believed made people able to do great things.

The involvement was not deliberate, but rather was sprung on me like a bear trap. It was reported in the paper that a high school student had committed suicide. What the article didn't say, and which I was advised of by someone within the school, was that he was part of a group that played D&D during activity time in the school. I was also told that the game might have been implicated in his suicide.

The game is a fantasy role playing game, where the players actually take on the roles of their characters, and some can identify so closely with these characters that they become them. In this game there is the conjuring up of spells and calling down of demons, witchcraft and sorcery.

After being goaded by some friends, I wrote a letter to the newspaper warning against kids playing fantasy role playing games, because it was shown to be dangerous for some who couldn't distinguish fantasy from reality. Out of nowhere I was then asked to debate with someone, who was in favor of these games, on the radio. After which I had reporters from TV and radio call to interview me. One thing it did give me was an inside view as to how the media sets you up. They'd come over to my office, and very nicely say, "I'm just going to ask you...," and supposedly would be giving you a heads up on what seemed to be a reasonable, fair and honest question. Then as soon as the cameras started to roll, they'd say, "How long have you been a hate-filled, intolerant, neo-Nazi, anti-abortion, Christian bigot?"

In researching this game I found many examples of kids across the nation getting so caught up with their own demons that they would physically act out the scenarios, and ended up killing themselves because they had a spell cast on them, or were told they would be killed. I saw this as a potential danger and brought these findings to the attention of the school board, and made the recommendation that this game should not be allowed as a sanctioned school activity as it may affect vulnerable students adversely.

One would expect that this would have been received by everyone as a reasonable concern and request and that they would look into it themselves. That was not the outcome. The firestorm that followed was, in my opinion, over the top. I was publicly accused of being a religious zealot and intolerant Nazi who wanted to strip away the cherished right of freedom to play any game the students wanted in school. (Now up till that time, I didn't think that was a right guaranteed by the Constitution, or that 14-15 year old students had any right to determine what they were allowed to do in school.)

I even arranged for experts and those with firsthand experience with this game to come to town and put on an informational night for those interested in learning more. They all agreed that vulnerable students were at risk.

Because of this, the editorial in the newspaper called me, among other things, "a member of the thought police," "the Ayatollah of Bedford" and "a book burner." They likened me to some of the most despised people in history, and deemed me likely mentally unstable. Just because I questioned the wisdom of young teens playing this game.

People even called the Pastor of the church I was going to and asked if he agreed with this madman, who was in his congregation, and was asked when he was going to denounce me. Luckily for me he said he did agree with me. Always good to have at least one man of God on your side.

I actually had patients call to have their medical records transferred to other physicians because of my stance on this. People who once talked to me in the hospital, now avoided me and any association with me. Well-meaning folks, who were still talking to me, couldn't understand why I would involve myself in this whole thing. I didn't know myself, but it was just something I felt called to do. If not me, who?

In the end, after a big dust up with people in town forming skirmish lines, the school board refused to take any action to disallow playing the game on school time. However, the teacher who oversaw the activity said he would no longer allow it because he didn't want to be responsible for what might happen. So de facto, the game ended in school.

When You Just Don't Fit In

One thing I should have known from the beginning is that I wouldn't be getting many, if any, patients from Richmond, Bedford Hill, Roxbury or the more desirable parts of town. I just didn't fit in well with the privileged elites. They were expecting special treatment, deference, and getting their own way. And then they would be shocked, I mean absolutely shocked, that you actually billed them for your services, which was not worth nearly as much as the time they spent waiting in your waiting room. In fact I should be paying them for having been able to kiss their ring and been granted an audience with them. I did much better with the middle class and the poor. And as Jesus said, "The poor you will always have with you," and we did and therefore, I never lacked for patients.

Nursing home rounds were made on my "day off." There were also rounds to be made at an elderly housing complex. Two old homes were converted, by a Lithuanian order of nuns, into elderly housing, one for men and the other for women. They named it the Villa St. Joseph. Whether this was because the Bible never mentions anything about St. Joseph getting old, or because the assumption is that, when St. Joseph died, he had Jesus and Mary at his bedside, was unclear. The villa was comprised of 2 very large, very old houses built around 1850. They were clapboard, as were most of the houses in the area, and two stories. On the first floor was the kitchen, with the stove, sink and refrigerator, a dining room with a table that seated 10, and a small sitting area with a couch, a love seat and a couple of side chairs. They also had the quarters for the nuns who ran the house tucked away on the side. On the second floor there were a couple of small bathrooms and 8 small bedrooms large enough for a single bed, a night stand, a small desk, a chair and the crucifix hanging on the wall. It was very monastery like. The stairs were made of wood, uncarpeted, and creaked with each step. The bannister was sturdy and made out of mahogany. The walls were papered with patterns from the 1950's, and the floors were worn wood.

By today's standards, the Villa would have been declared a major fire trap, and would never be allowed to operate. Anyone caught upstairs with a fire on the first floor would never be able to get down. They did put fire escape ladders on some of the outside second floor windows, but most of these folks would have killed themselves trying to get down them. But since there were no candles, no smoking, no open flames and no fires, everyone was content.

The nuns from this order all came from Lithuania, via Canada, and the residents were all Lithuanian, having come from parts unknown. Many were known to have escaped from Communist persecution in their homeland. In order to be accepted to live in the home, you had to have mobility, and your wits about you. There were stairs they were required to climb to get to the upper floor rooms, where all the bedrooms were. And then they had to be able to get down the stairs to get to the dining room, where they had their meals. This was staffed and run by 3 nuns, who lived on site. They asked me if I would be the doctor for their residents, which I was pleased to do. Not knowing how to speak Lithuanian was a big drawback, but as long as I had an interpreter, I was OK. Sister Palmera was the nun in charge. If a patient had a problem, instead of calling me, she had her own Lithuanian folk remedies that she would try on them. If they refused to get better after her ministrations, then she'd call me in as a consultant.

Sister Palmira was a big advocate of outdoor exercise for old folks. She herself would go on 5-10 mile hikes all around, and encouraged the residents to go for walks as well. One elderly lady took her advice, and went for a walk in the wooded area around the house and never came back. When she didn't show up for dinner, they sent out the search party. When they found her, she said she got "lost in the forest," and couldn't find her way out. After that, if they were going out for exercise, they had to bring someone else with them, and preferably someone without dementia.

Sister Olivet was the administrator. She had to decide when someone was no longer capable of this independent living arrangement. It usually became self-evident when that person either fell down the stairs, or needed oxygen and a nitro pill after they went up.

Sister Clair was a very young woman, and would probably have been considered the intern. She had some very traumatic experiences growing up. When I went over to the Villa, I would sometimes spend more time with Sister Clair than with the residents. Apparently, the order of nuns wasn't quite sure she was nun material, and were pressuring her to leave the order. Like the Navy Seals, all she had to do was ring the bell, and they would let up on her, and she would be free to go. They were concerned that she was "escaping her problems by going into the convent." They kept telling her that God had something else in mind for her, but she couldn't see it and was really scared to live outside the convent. This was later proved to be true. In the end, she did leave the order and married a man, who truly loved her, and was devoted to her. It appeared God did have other plans for her. She was released from a convent life to be a loving wife and mother.

These Lithuanian nuns also had a convent, as well as a full-fledged nursing home, for those who could not get around, or did not have their wits about them. It was at that nursing home that I had an odd experience. A patient's daughter and son-in-law wanted to interview me before choosing a physician for their mother. Her mother was a bright, alert, oriented and very pleasant lady. They were moving her out of their town, and from a neighboring state. When I sat down with them, the first question they asked was if I enjoyed taking care of geriatric patients. After passing that test, the real reason for the interview and the transfer was made known. "What is your philosophy of treating an elderly patient at the end of life?" It turned out that the nursing home the patient was at previously was run by a physician whose cultural norms were different from the ones we are used to in our country. This patient had become sick with an infection. The family, who had been visiting the patient, asked why she was not being treated. The physician told her, "She's old. She's going to die sooner or later anyway. Why waste medical resources on her? Just let her die. That's the way we do it in my country." After she told him in no uncertain terms, "Well, that's not the way we do it in this country, and I will not let you do that to my mother," she pulled her mother out of that nursing home and brought her to the local ER and then to the Lithuanian nursing home.

It was incidents like this that made me wonder about how the value of life had changed. When I was in medical school to be called an abortionist was about the worst thing you could call a doctor. Now abortions are not only allowed, they are even encouraged, and the abortionists are celebrated as heroes of the women's rights and choice crowd. Where would this lead? It seems to lead to abortions for any and all reasons, even for sex selection, and at any and all times during the pregnancy, or in some cases, even after the birth.

It also seems to lead us to allow the frail and elderly to "quietly slip away," or maybe even help them along if they're not quick enough about it.

CHAPTER 9

Our New Office

It seemed that, with the practice being a success, we'd be staying the rest of our working lives in Bainbridge. With this in mind I decided I would try to find some land, and build a new office for myself with some room for expansion. After searching around the area, it became clear that finding the right place was not going to be easy. The lawyer for the city of Bainbridge wanted me to locate my office in one of the abandoned Montgomery Ward Department store buildings in the center of town. Unfortunately, as I told him, there was no parking, and the patients would have to get to the 2nd floor in a building without an elevator. A lot of renovation would have to be done to make it work, and for which, he felt, I should be financially responsible.

Those selling commercial real estate wanted to sell large tracts of land, which required a lot of site work, and which was financially out of reach for me. One particularly large and difficult tract would one day contain a McDonald's, a Subway restaurant, a bank and a number of other commercial stores. By not purchasing that land the opportunity for me to make a fortune in real-estate was lost.

When we did find a good location with land for sale, which seemed to be reasonably priced, we bought it, trusting the real-estate salesman. After we purchased it, we found out it had some problems. The first of which was that the land was a dump site after a flood 30 years ago. The old houses, which were destroyed by the flood, were dumped on to this site and then buried. When we did some borings, we discovered that, on parts of the land, there was wood underneath which was still decaying and making the land unstable for building upon. In fact, we could only build on one corner of the property—the corner on which we didn't want to put the building. But we would make it work.

The second problem was that it was still zoned for residential use, even though it was on a major road into the city. We had to go for a zone change before we could proceed. Because it was residential, they would not allow driveway access onto the major road, stating that the "sight lines" were not adequate (even though one could see ½ a mile down the road in either direction).

The third problem was that half the land was in the city of Bainbridge and half was in the town of Bainbridge. While that didn't seem like a problem before we bought the land, it ended up making everything much more complicated. We had to get the town **and** the city, with their 2 separate boards, to agree to change the zone. Plus we were taxed twice, once by the town and again by the city, on the same building. Even though we paid a tax for the fire department in the city, we also had to pay one for the town fire department.

Providentially, Glen, a man I met through the Rotary Club and who also became a friend as well as a patient, was on the zoning boards, and guided the process through for us. They eventually gave us street access, and zoned the whole area commercial. This eventually allowed for other doctor's offices to be built on the same road, how convenient.

Practice Philosophy

It was about this time that I really began to see the importance of addressing, and taking care of, not just the physical, but the mental, emotional and spiritual health of my patients. The spiritual aspect really focused on the issue of their faith. It was not really a question of whether they had a particular religious belief. Rather it was to assess if they had any spiritual aspect to their lives—what they believed and trusted in when things went bad. Did they have a supportive or faith community? What gave their life meaning and purpose? What gave them hope? Were they prepared to handle death, theirs or their loved ones'? Some patients had a very difficult time with some of these questions. Some felt they were seeing a doctor to "take care of my body and leave my soul alone, thank you." Others welcomed the questions and were grateful for the opportunity to share their beliefs, worries and concerns.

Some folks had the idea that their faith would prevent bad things from happening to them. When some catastrophic event occurred, their faith was severely challenged. They needed to know that faith was not a magic amulet, used to ward off evil. It was to carry them through when nothing else could. Sometimes God cures us and sometimes He weeps and mourns and grieves with us. Some losses, such as the death of a child or the death of a spouse, are particularly severe. The grief from these never truly goes away. You don't just get over it, no matter how much faith you have or how much time goes by. You just learn how to live with the hope you will be reunited in a better place where there is no longer death and sorrow in the future.

I would inquire of my patients if they had a religious affiliation, and if critically ill, would they would want me to call a priest or minister for them. (This was before hospital chaplains.) Once when I asked a man, who claimed to be Catholic, if he would want me to call a priest to give him the sacrament of the sick, he said, "Do I need to worry, Doc? Are you trying to tell me something? Is it bad?"

We named our practice St. Luke's Family Practice for a couple of reasons. First, Luke, the writer of the Gospel, was a physician. Second, we wanted people to know that the faith component was important to the health of a person. I have seen people take their first breath and their last breath. And I noticed that their physical health was affected by their spiritual, emotional and mental health. The most important words they needed to hear or say were "I love you,"

"I'm sorry, please forgive me," "I forgive you" and "Thank you for all you've done for me." These words healed better than antibiotics.

In a way, the practice was founded on faith, the faith of my father. During my time in medical school, my dad would stop at churches during his driving time for work, and pray to St. Jude, the patron saint of hopeless cases, and light candles. Maybe I wasn't hopeless but I certainly needed all the help I could get. In gratitude, we put up a small statue of St. Jude my father gave me and a plaque of St. Luke my uncle gave me

Peter

Rev. Peter Ellington was a retired Episcopal priest. He would fill in when the pastor was away or needed a break. He was a chaplain in WWII, and was sent into combat with the troops. He said that when he signed up for the military, he didn't think that the chaplains would actually be in combat, so it was a surprise to him when he began experiencing the Germans shelling his position. He said his first thought at that time was, "What in the world am I doing here?" Fortunately or unfortunately, his combat experience was cut short when the lower portion of his left leg was blown off by a shell exploding next to him. From then on, Peter had an ongoing relationship with the VA hospital.

Peter and I would have long discussions about his experiences and theology. I was becoming very interested in theology, and as Peter was a former teacher in a seminary, and clergyman, I thought he could answer my inquiries, and he enjoyed the discussions. Peter was always good natured, jovial and had a very calming presence, which is good to have if you are in the clergy business, even though he spent most of his time writing books and teaching at school, rather than pastoring.

He would joke, when talking about "faith healers" doing miracles. He didn't believe in them or in those TV preachers promising miracles for a "love offering." He said he had the "acid test" of their ability, and would knock on his wooden leg. "If they can heal this, then I'll believe in them."

Peter gave very folksy sermons, and was always self-deprecating, even though he was very intelligent and had a professorial background. I got to know him over many years and, as he was getting on in age, he noticed the deterioration of his body. In his younger years, he was a brilliant man, who wrote many books and commentaries, which made his aging process even more difficult for him. He was acutely aware of what functions he was losing almost daily.

During one visit, the conversation turned to his death, and what it would be like. I asked him what he would ask Jesus upon meeting Him in heaven. My thought in asking him this was to find out what great mystery of God he would like to know about. For someone so learned, I expected him to ask for an explanation of the Trinity or just how the bread and wine became the body and blood of Christ or why God allows pain and suffering.

He thought for a moment, as he always did, and then said, "I think I would ask Him, if I got any of it right," meaning "did I teach and understand any of the faith correctly?"

"What do you think Jesus would say?" I asked.

"You came close, a couple of times," he replied. I interpreted that to mean he would be disappointed to have lived his life for Christ, and to have missed the whole point.

I thought about his answer and said, "Peter, if we need to get it right, I mean to really understand God and His message perfectly, who would be able to be saved?"

Peter thought for about a minute and then said, "That's why He sent Jesus, so He could get it right for us. I guess we just need to trust Him. That should suffice, shouldn't it?"

"And you trust Him?"

"Yes I do."

"Well, then 'Well done good and faithful servant,'" I said.

"But wouldn't you really like to know?"

"Yeah, I guess we all would."

Harold

It was in the summer that I first met Harold, when he was brought to the ER with severe shortness of breath. Being on medical service, I was called in to admit him to the hospital. When I first saw him, it was obvious that he had severe lung disease from his cigarette smoking, and was in an extremely critical condition. He was an emaciated man in his early 60's sitting in the bed bolt upright with an oxygen mask on his face and gasping for air. But his condition didn't preclude his disdain for everyone who was there to help him. He had no medical insurance, and didn't want to answer any questions regarding his medical history or his next of kin. He said he was entitled to medical care without having to put up with the 3rd degree. He kept asking for a cigarette, and was quite vocal with slurs and curses when the staff nurse wouldn't give him one. His attitude didn't endear him to anyone having to take care of him. He seemed to be bitter, had a chip on his shoulder and was just itching for a fight or argument.

Looking at his lab tests, it seemed that this night might be his last, so I felt the need to talk to him about the possibility of his dying. I asked if he had any religious beliefs, if he believed in God, or went to any particular church, or maybe would like a chaplain or priest. Harold said that he didn't think God existed. When asked why, he said that if God did exist, he would not allow all the suffering to go on, especially the way some people treated others so cruelly. It turned he was talking about how cruelly he had been treated over his lifetime. His father was abusive to him. He was told to get out of the house when he was 15 years old and made to fend for himself. His mother, who was also beaten by her husband, just cowered in the corner.

He joined the Navy, lying about his age and got into trouble almost immediately for insubordination. It seemed he had a very difficult time taking orders from anyone in authority. After spending some time in the brig, he was dishonorably discharged and spent the rest of his life hanging out with petty criminals and helping them with their petty crimes: mostly breaking and entering, robbery, felonies and the occasional assault and battery. The police knew him well. He had developed a hatred for people who were white or wealthy in his eyes, and felt they should share their wealth with people like him, who had very little.

Eventually after his associates tried to kill him for taking more that his "fair share" from a job they did together, he fled and ended up doing odd jobs, janitorial work or occasional farm work. He ended up in our town because of the mills and thought he could get a job there, and did until he could no longer do the work because of his medical condition.

I didn't expect a discussion of why God does things or allows things. I told him, "I don't know why people treat others so badly, but I do know that it's written that God sent his own son to become a man on this earth, and as I remember, we didn't treat him very well either. As the story goes, they put Him on a cross. And even though they did that to him, it says He still loves us and wants to forgive and save us. I don't know why God does that either. If it were me I'd incinerate the whole place, and that would include you and me. Do we deserve any better after what we've done?"

Harold just smiled, and said, "Do you have a Bible I could read?" I got a Gideon Bible from in the room, and brought it to him. He didn't die that night, and he remained my patient. Harold told me later that it was that night, for the first time, he saw himself as not only the victim of cruelty, but also as a perpetrator. He said it was a revelation to him.

Since Harold was a black man, and at the time it was the new vogue to refer to him as African-American, I asked him how he wanted to be described. He said, “I’ve been called colored, negro and black, but I don’t understand this African-American thing. I’ve never been to Africa. Why would they call me African?” So I just called him a friend.

One day Harold came in complaining that his feet were hurting.

“How long have your feet been hurting?” I asked.

“Oh, since I jumped out of a window and broke my feet.”

“Jumped out of a window! When did you jump out a window?”

“About 30 years ago,” he said thinking back.

“How high up were you?”

“Two stories up.”

“What in the world would possess you to jump out of a second story window? Was the building on fire?”

“Well,” he said, “I was with this girl, and her husband was coming in the door, and the window was the only way out. And I sure didn’t want to meet him ‘cause I didn’t know if he had a gun.”

Trying to moralize, I asked if she was worth breaking both his feet for a sexual indiscretion.

“Oh, yeah, she was.”

So much for moralizing.

Bert came in as a new patient one summer. Bert was a 35 year old man. When I asked him why he had come in, he said he just wanted a check-up. He had previously been very heavily into drugs and wanted to have his blood checked to make sure nothing was showing up from his past habits. When I asked him how long he had been clean, he said about 15 years. "How did you kick it?" I asked.

Bert said something happened to him that changed his life. It seemed he was into alcohol, drugs and all the generally well known self-destructive behaviors that one would be able to get into. Because of this, he was involved in a serious auto accident while on one of his alcohol binges. He described the incident in a very vivid way. At first he was reluctant to share it. He didn't think I would believe him or might think he was crazy. He said he never told anyone else about it, but he eventually related it.

He said that immediately after the accident, he seemed to wake up in a very dark place. He said, "Imagine the very blackest black that you could imagine. It was darker than that."

While he was in the blackness, he felt there was something, or someone, next to him that was even blacker than the black surroundings. He said the only way he could describe this other being was as something indescribably frightening and evil. Even though, at the time, he did not believe in a hell or a devil, he said he was terrified.

"All I could do was to get down on my knees and pray, 'Please, God, save me' over and over again. Now understand, I didn't even know if I believed in God." While doing this he could hear the voice of the being next to him, telling him it was too late for that.

Then suddenly, he said, he saw an angel, all in white, and extremely bright, coming toward him. He interrupted his story at this point to ask, "Do you know why when angels present themselves to humans in the Bible they always start out saying 'Fear not'? Because they are huge. They are big and powerful and frightening!"

When this angel appeared, he heard the dark creature next to him say, "Stay away from him, he's mine. He's mine. It's too late for you." He said it was a voice that made him shudder.

But the angel said, "Get away from him, Satan, it's not his time. He's got to go back."

After hearing this, he woke up in the wrecked car with his chest crushed, his limbs broken, and in severe pain. If he survived all the injuries, he promised God he would clean up his life, and live a life pleasing to God, which he had done for the last 15 years.

Some people would contend that what Bert experienced was a hallucination, perhaps brought on by his drugs, or something imagined and not real. In fact Bert wonders about that himself. But you could never get Bert to deny that what he had experienced was very real to him. Real enough to get him off his drugs and change his life totally.

Bert was working as an aide in a facility for disabled adults, so he needed to have himself checked for TB and other infectious diseases on a routine basis. As it turned out, Bert's lab work showed that his liver tests were elevated and with further evaluation, it turned up he had contracted Hepatitis C.

I knew that this would not go over well with his employer. So I called him back to tell him the bad news. Bert said that when he turned in that report, he would be fired from his job because it required patient contact. And there was no other job there that didn't involve patient contact.

Bert was devastated. He couldn't understand how, after all these years of being clean and trying to do what was right, this would happen. "Was God punishing me now, after all these years for something that I did so long ago?" he wanted to know.

I really didn't know what to say to him. I can't answer for God. "I don't think God is really interested in punishing you for what you did. He's more interested in wanting to save you," I said. "I think nature and the natural consequences of what you did are just catching up to you. And for that you need to get treated. I'm going to refer you to a specialist for this. As far as God goes, I would recommend you talk with your pastor, priest or minister. He may have a better answer than I have for you."

Bert was fired and was devastated. He went for treatment and eventually got another job as a custodian in a large church in the city, where a pastor heard about his plight and hired him. He wasn't making as much money, but at least he had a job and people around him who cared about him.

CHAPTER 10

The Recruit

The successive nights without sleep and the lack of family time had taken its toll on me, so after 5 years I finally decided to hire another doctor to practice with me. I had just built the new office building and thought this getting out of bed in the darkest hours of the night would be best shared with someone. In order to get a doctor for the summer one had to begin advertising in winter or, the latest, early spring.

Many folks think that hiring another doctor should be a fairly easy thing to do. But the fact was that one had to recruit, and entice someone to come and work with you. Ads had to be placed in the journals, and they had to be creative. How many docs would look at an ad for "Long hours for very little pay, located in one of the least desirable places in the state, with shopping available 1 hour away and the lovely smell of cow manure year round, but balanced off by high taxes and a high cost of living" and say, "That's just the place I was looking for!" So I had to take a little poetic license to have the slightest chance that anyone would contact me to inquire about the position. So my ad read: "Great place to raise a family (meaning: low murder rate), good schools (well, maybe not great, but there were some private schools within driving distance), shopping nearby (nearby is a very relative term), lovely patient population (when they wanted to be, and if you weren't looked upon as a foreigner), top tier hospital (if top tier meant open and accepting patients) and able to make a good (relative term again) living." That worked until they showed up and said, "Where's the place you mentioned in your ad?"

Luckily for me a doc, who had family in the state and who had just come off a mission location in some desolate Caribbean Island, came to visit. Our town looked like downtown Manhattan to him. There was actually drinkable water, a variety of foods you didn't have to pick off a tree, no roaches in your rice and no scorpions in your shoes. It was a relatively easy sell.

The only problem, initially, was he was still on Caribbean time. He took a siesta every day, enjoyed a bottle of vino, and had a *manana* attitude. Everything was *hakuna matata.* I, being a type A personality, had to have everything done yesterday, and the bill collectors did not have this *hakuna matata* philosophy. As the weather got colder, I gave him more responsibility for the running of the practice, and the conflict between *hakuna matata* and meeting payroll became evident, and the siestas stopped. In the end, everything worked out well.

Choosing a Church

Choosing a church in our town was a fairly significant decision. It was the kind of town where what church you attended determined who your closest friends would be, your social status, and what the others in town thought of you. You were also expected to patronize the businesses and stores run by the people in your congregation.

In my view (which may not be totally accurate, so don't take this as gospel), the way it broke down was like this. The Episcopal Church people were generally known for their being the most affluent folks in town. Although most of their money was inherited, they did own most of the factories and larger businesses. They were known for their cocktail parties, Christmas craft sales and liberal ideas, such as the first to accept women and homosexuals as pastors. As one member expressed it, "The great thing about this church is that you can believe in anything and still be a member," and that about summed it up.

The Lutheran Church people had a strong German background and were hard working folks. They owned the butcher shop, the pasty and pie shop, and were known for their Old World costumes, bratwurst and beer at their Oktoberfest each fall. They were conservative politically and theologically, and were the last hold outs to not accept modern worship music and praise songs. "The altar is nowhere to put a keyboard, a drum set and a guitar stand. If the organ was good enough for Martin Luther to use, then it should be good enough for us" was there philosophy. Then again, they accepted all new-fangled ideas slowly. After all it was only during World War II that they decided to have the services only in English instead of German. Some people would call them backward in their ideas, but they preferred the term traditional.

The Catholic Church mainly consisted of folks from French-Canadian heritage. They had their bingo, their fundraising and led the St. Patrick's Day celebrations with the yearly raffle for a brand new car, donated by Gagne Motors. They also ran the Catholic Elementary school, taught by the Sisters of St. Anne, whose students, it seemed, were always fundraising. There was the chocolate bar sale, the magazine sale, the fruit sale, the greeting card sale, the fruitcake sale and the yard sale. Most folks in the community bought into at least one of these. The Catholic Church was a contradiction to some folks. They were liberal in their thinking when it came to social issues—against the death penalty, for taking care of the homeless and in favor of strong labor unions—but very conservative in other issues—against abortion, against women ordination and against priests marrying. And while they were strong on Papal or clerical authority, on novenas, on lighting candles, on all things Mary, on doing good works and on fundraising for causes, they were short on Bible study. But they did have a catechism that told you everything you needed to know about getting into heaven.

The Methodist Church mainly consisted of refugees from the Episcopal Church, who didn't feel they fit in because their financial status was not up to par. They were known for, and spent most of their time on, collecting food for food banks and clothes for thrift shops. The Methodists were definitely Social Gospel folks. While the Lutherans would sometimes chide the Methodists about trying to earn their way into heaven, they knew that without the Methodists, the town would be a much harder place to live for those without means. They also tended to be quite liberal in their thinking about abortions, women in the clergy and in their interpretation of Scripture. "You can't believe everything that's in there, you know," they would say.

The Presbyterian Church had by far the most intellectually driven people. They loved reading Calvin's Institutes and the Westminster Confession along with Scripture. They had it all figured out and if you didn't agree with them, they'd be happy to spend the next 6 hours convincing you why they were right. They had the most rigorous Sunday school classes in town. Those classes were not for socializing. They were there to learn, and they were the only Sunday school classes that had a syllabus, and assigned homework each week. You may have even been able to parlay some of those classes into a seminary degree. They may not have been the jolliest of folks, but they were certainly the most self-assured. Of the folks who were Presbyterian, many were of English and Scottish background, so they would sponsor the highland games and haggis festival every year. But because no one could stomach the haggis, they substituted a chowder fest instead, but they kept the name as a tradition.

The Congregationalist Church was by far the most liberal, theologically speaking. They were the most inclusive. You didn't have to believe in Jesus or be a Christian in their view. They had their share of Buddhists, Hindus and Unitarians. Their motto was "As long as you believe in something, you'll be fine." They were not strong in doctrinal purity except the one that said "if you had doctrinal purity, you were wrong." Their big event was having a 4th of July Jamboree, which included a tag sale, a chicken barbeque, a cake walk and music by the coronet band. They felt that the 4th of July was sufficiently secular so as not to take sides on anything theological nor to offend any religion.

The Baptist Church and Evangelical church was strong on Bible study and teaching sermons, but weak on sacraments. To me going to church on Sunday and not having the Lord's Supper was like going to a restaurant and only getting the appetizer and not the main meal. And they didn't believe in baptizing infants. To which the question was raised: What about original sin? How do you deal with that? Their answer was that there was no such thing. Rather there was an inherited propensity to sin. Children didn't sin until they were old enough to know they were sinning. So it appeared, from that belief, that Jesus was not the only one born without sin. We are all born without sin. They also were big on working out your salvation, but in contrast with some other denominations, they worked it out by making mission trips, supporting missionaries, and evangelizing your neighbor. How many converts you made was important. If you could get someone to accept Jesus Christ as their Lord and Savior, even for just an instance, that would count as a win. Lack of perseverance in the faith was not counted against you.

So choosing a church was a significant event for Maria and me after coming to town. We were raised Roman Catholic, but were attracted by a church with strong Bible study and convictions. But churches that had those qualities were not the ones with a liturgical service and the tradition of the Sacraments, especially the Baptism of infants and the Communion, which we preferred.

We looked at all the churches in town and immediately ruled out the Catholic Church due to authority issues. The Episcopal Church had some attraction at the beginning. They did have the Sacraments and some Bible studies. The only problem was Father Boyd. Father Boyd studied in a seminary that looked at the Bible from a historical and naturalistic perspective. So, from his point of view, when it said that Jesus fed 5000 with 5 loaves and 2 fish, what it really meant is that everyone shared their food with each other so there was plenty to go around. Or if it said that Jesus rose from the dead, since we all know that people really don't come back from the dead, it meant that His spirit came back and the Apostles remembered Him as He was.

That was a brook too far to cross for us. For us the Bible "says what it means and means what it says." If it says He walked on water, then by God, He walked on water. Don't come up with any stories about His knowing where the big rocks were.

While I was attending the Episcopal church I went on a retreat weekend that changed my life. I came home excited about my faith and wanted to share this experience with everyone. I told Father Boyd about it and his response was classic, "Don't worry. You'll get over it. This too will pass." But I said, "I don't want to get over it. I want it to last."

The Presbyterians were very nice folks, but the idea that God would chose some for salvation and then chose some for damnation, just didn't feel right. Even though we did agree with the Presbyterians, that truth is not based on feelings, we could never get on board with TULIP, the acronym for their belief. In our mind God wanted no one to be lost and Christ died for all, not just for a select number.

We talked to the Methodists, who saw us as more workers drones for their food bank and clothing store. We seemed to be taking part in what seemed to be more of a job interview than a church membership. I was busy enough with my practice and Maria with our kids. We didn't think we wanted to take on another job at that point.

The First Baptist and the Free Evangelical Church were also rejected. We knew that to join the Baptist church we would need to be re-baptized. However, according to the Creed, we believed there was only one Baptism needed and we'd had it.

The Good News Free Evangelical Church had a great Sunday school program and a good youth program. Initially we started going there, and the kids learned their Bible. But in the end, it was their lack of sacraments that ended it for us. Their not really wanting to baptize children, their not believing in weekly communion nor in the "Real Presence" at communion and their "once saved always saved philosophy" didn't seem to agree with Scripture. Also the idea that all women had to wear long dresses when out in public, all children were to be home schooled and no drinking of alcoholic beverages was a bit more than we thought necessary for salvation. Even though we did like the idea of long dresses and home schooling the kids, and actually did talk about that, we didn't want to be in a group that made it mandatory.

Finally we spoke with Pastor Bauer of the Lutheran Church. The Lutherans had Sacraments, which I liked, and also had a high view of Scripture, which Maria liked. So in the end we elected to become Lutherans.

It was only after we were investigating the Lutheran Church did we find that there are 2 common branches of the Church, the ELCA and the LCMS. We attended an ELCA church and after the service I stopped and asked the pastor, "What's the difference between the ELCA and the LCMS?" He told me, "Oh, those LCMS people, they actually believe the Bible is true." I felt that was as good an endorsement as any to join the LCMS Lutherans.

But Do You Believe It?

Theology had always interested me, especially how to reconcile all the Bible stories, particularly Old Testament stories, with the science that I had studied. The Creation of man vs. Darwin's evolution, the Genesis flood story, Jonah and the whale and many others.

During medical school I got to know and talk to Pastor Jim Danelley, who actually believed the Bible to be true. Not all pastors or ministers actually believed that. One Easter Sunday, during my training, I had attended a church service and heard a wonderful sermon on the resurrection of Christ, and what it means to us today. After the service I got to talking to the minister over lunch, and told him I was training to be a doctor. "Oh," said the minister, "so you're a man of science. Do you believe in the resurrection of Christ?" "Yes, I think I do." (I never really had to pick a side on that one before.) "Your sermon today certainly points me to believe that it's true."

"Well, that's good," said the minister. "I wish I could believe it."

"You don't believe it?" I was shocked. "How could you deliver such a good sermon about the resurrection, if you don't believe it's true?"

"It's the job. You do what you have to do to make a living. You see for me it was either be a social worker or a minister. I chose to be a minister. The job is very similar, except I felt the ministry carried more authority over those I would be counseling. Don't get me wrong. I do believe that Jesus lived and died. I think he was a good man with a lot of good ideas, like Buddha or Gandhi. He showed us how we should live. But the miracles and the resurrection is just too much to believe as true. Myth, fable, maybe."

That conversation stuck with me. If this minister, who studied all about this in seminary, didn't believe in the Bible, why should I? It was at that point, I had to get to the truth of the whole matter. If I was to believe in all this theology stuff, it had to be because it was true, not because I wished it was true. I had to be convinced, especially since I was raising children in this faith. I didn't want my kids to find out at some point that God, like Santa Claus or the Easter Bunny, was just made up by the adults in their lives.

This led me on a quest to find out. I read C.S. Lewis, John Stott, J.I. Packer and others, but I needed to talk to someone, who believed in this, about my questions. That's how I got involved with talking to Jim Danelley.

I talked with Jim for hours. We would sometime meet for lunch or in the evenings. I would present all the scientific theories, and Jim would try, with little success to adequately answer those objections to the Bible accounts. Then one day, after I presented the latest argument against Jonah, Jim simply said, "OK, that's all fine. But it really all comes down to one question, which only you can answer. What about Jesus? Who do you think He is? Because that is the question that really divides the believers from the non-believers. It matters little whether Jonah lived. But it is of great importance if Jesus lived. It is of great importance if he died and then rose from the dead. It is of great importance if he really was God as he claimed to be. These are the questions you have to come to terms with. These are the questions you'll need to answer, and which will determine, according to the Bible, where you spend eternity."

That exchange caught me by surprise. I thought the Bible and Jesus were all in the same bag. If you believed in the Bible, you believed in Jesus. But Jim was indicating it really was the other way round. If you believed in Jesus, then He was the One who validated the Bible as true. So now the questions all revolved around this Jesus and who He was or who He thought He was. Was Jesus an actual historical figure or just a myth? It turned out that there were other sources other than the Bible, which spoke of Him and documented that He actually lived.

But the greatest single issue, upon which the whole argument either stood or fell, in my mind, was the resurrection. Did He actually rise from the dead, bodily? Can this be proven to be true without a shadow of a doubt? Can we know for sure? I was looking for evidence. The Bible account alone didn't offer enough proof for me. The story could have been made up.

Jim argued that Jesus' body was never produced by His enemies, the Romans or the Jewish leaders. This simple thing would have been enough to discredit His followers who were going around proclaiming that they saw Him alive again after His death and burial. It didn't happen. Still not enough for me though. Lots of people believe things and even see things that aren't true.

"But the Apostles died for what they believed," said Jim.

"Lots of people die for what they believe to be true. That doesn't make what they believe true. They just think it's true."

But the convincing argument was: "People will die for something that they **think** is true. But no one will die a slow and painful death for something they know is absolutely not true. If Christ did not rise from the grave, the Apostles surely would have known. When the swords came out, and they had to die for this story they were telling, their persistence flies in the face of all reason. They surely would not have died for a story that they made up, and knew was false. It was their testimonies and deaths that convinced others that Jesus had actually risen from the dead. It is His resurrection that the church was founded on. Now what do you believe about Jesus? Do you have enough assurance that He rose from the dead? Do you believe He is who He said He is—the Son of God? Do you believe He died for your sins? Do you trust that through His death your sins were forgiven? Do you put your faith and trust in Him? Who do you trust with your eternal life? Because in the end, that's all that matters."

His questions were relentless, but right on the mark. It was at that point I went from a skeptical, possible believer to an all-out believer. I saw that it wasn't what you believed that was the most important, it was Who you believed in. It's not putting all your trust in a specific book or a specific church that claims to speak for God. It's putting all your trust in Him. It seemed so simple yet so profound. How could I have missed this for so many years?

Then I wrestled with the idea of man being created in the image of God. If man evolved from animals, then man was of no more value than an animal. If that is so, why do we consider it a crime to kill a human, but not to hunt and kill a deer? It must be because man has God's image and an animal doesn't. And why does man have a feeling of guilt after doing something he knows is wrong? Why do men have consciences? Animals certainly don't. Why are humans the only animal able to question their own programing and their own nature and natural desires? Why do all men, from all times in history, have a code of acceptable conduct? And when that code is broken, why do they appeal to a justice and fairness that is outside of themselves, and above themselves, and binding on everyone and which everyone is to obey? This can only be there because God put it there. For me the matter was settled.

CHAPTER 11

In the Classroom

I became involved in talking to the 5th grades in an attempt to keep them from becoming smokers. A big part of the presentation was warning the kids about peer pressure. How their peers could pressure them into doing something dumb. I noted that all boys at their age have a very difficult time refusing a dare, especially if someone is calling them "chicken." "A dare is an invitation to do something you will regret, and a double dog dare is usually an invitation to the Emergency room." To prove my point, I said, "I bet if I dared all the boys to run up to the roof, and jump off, half the class would head up to the roof." At this point, if there were no teachers to stop them, half the boys would be out of the classroom and finding the nearest stairways.

Another time, a particular school wanted me to give the presentation to all 5 fifth grade classes, all 120 students, at once in the auditorium. Even though I tried to explain that this program was meant for small classes and student interaction, the teachers wouldn't budge. It was their way or no way. So I said I would try. The presentation was like a circus. Kids were talking, poking, punching each other, getting up, changing chairs, and acting like wild chimpanzees while generally ignoring me as best they could. The teachers were correcting papers, reading books, completing crossword puzzles and all the while ignoring the chaotic situation, and making no attempt to gain control over the pandemonium of the students. At one point in the presentation, I would ask the kids to give me adjectives to describe something. At this school the kids didn't know what adjectives were. So as I was apt to do, I said, as an aside talking to myself, in a low voice, "Oh, I forgot this is a public school." (Of course, the implication taken was you don't know anything because you're not getting an adequate education. And your teachers are terrible.) The teachers, who were generally snoozing and ignoring the entire presentation, suddenly woke up, and got incensed. It was absolutely amazing. They couldn't seem to hear the kids screaming at their friends on the other side of the auditorium, but that comment, said in a low voice, they heard loud and clear. And that school, of course, never let me back in to give another presentation. I thought, "It's a good thing I don't have to go there again. I'd probably have to bring a whip and cages the next time."

Decisions Have Consequences

Kathy came in to see me with an "embarrassing" problem. I had taken care of her medical needs since she was a baby, and I knew Kathy and her parents very well. As she got into high school, I began having "the talks" about not being led to do something by some boy, she would forever regret. When she was 15, she came in for an office visit complaining of a problem "down there." After examining her, I asked if she had had sexual relations. She reluctantly told me she had. "Why? Kathy, didn't we talk about that?" "Yes, but he told me he loved me. And it was my one and only time."

Then I had to tell her the news. She had not one, but two STDs for which she would need treatment. Luckily they were treatable. Sometimes we need to learn lessons painfully. I asked if she was still going out with him. She said, "No, he left me for another girl." "That's good for you but not for his new girlfriend. You might want to tell her to get checked out." It was cases like these that made me so passionate about talking to the teens in the junior high and high schools. I hated to see them getting taken advantage of. If I could have them avoid these situations, I thought it would be worth the effort and loss of a day's work.

My moral value system was tilting to the extreme right in comparison to the general mores of the day. There was no way to save these teens from making disastrous mistakes, if they didn't know they were making disastrous decisions in the first place. One bad decision at the right (or wrong, as you may view it) time, could impact them for the rest of their lives. Some just plain didn't want to be saved from making bad decisions. They thought there just was no fun in living life without taking life threatening risks. My mission was to make sure they were not ignorant as to what the perils and pitfalls were out there for them. So if they did make bad choices, they did so knowingly, and it was their willful and deliberate decision to do so. There was nothing anyone could really do about that.

There came the opportunity to talk at different venues as the polar opposite viewpoint of Planned Parenthood, which was always being invited to speak. The Planned Parenthood view was as long as no one got hurt, as long as everyone was OK with it, as long as "protection" was used (or abortion was utilized if it failed or wasn't used at all), everything was permissible. Because of the conservative, pro-life and abstinence label that was placed on me, I was invited to speak at high and junior high schools as the "fair and balanced" position, but only if I were invited by a student or a specific health teacher. One junior high school teacher asked me to speak to his classes on "not having sex until your married," or from the teacher's viewpoint, "not having sex at least until you're out of my class." They were pretty tired of having kids come to school pregnant. So the topic I spoke on was "How to find your true love."

Another teacher asked me to speak to her 9th grade health classes every year on avoiding STD's. I quickly found that the reason there was a problem in the first place was the students had no moral values or foundation upon which these kinds of moral decisions would be based. So my talks became 2 day marathons entitled, "How to find true happiness," and "How to not destroy your life." Other titles could also have been, "Why you should have integrity," or "Why do you want to go to such lengths to mess up your life," or "The one thing you don't want to happen to you will happen, unless you make sure it doesn't."

In doing this I found that the students were much more knowledgeable about the intimate details of their favorite entertainer or movie star, than they were with the 10 Commandments. (I mean who would have known that lying, cheating, dishonesty, sexual promiscuity, hatred, envy and greed were all bad things? What a revelation!) Money, pleasure seeking, power and fame were their gods, which was totally understandable since their role models and heroes also worshiped the same gods. This is where taking kids out of Sunday morning Sunday school and putting them into Sunday morning sports programs lead!

This is where I was learning that curing a kid's sore throat, suturing a laceration, setting a broken bone or sprained ankle, and then sending him back out with the same ideas that lying, cheating, stealing and taking advantage of others are all just means to an end, was not really treating them. I was only treating their short term illness, while ignoring the long term ones.

Going to Court

I was subpoenaed to testify in court by the attorney of a patient of mine who had MS and was seeking more financial assistance from her ex-husband, who divorced her after she got her diagnosis. She said that with the increasing disability, she needed more money to cover medical and other expenses. I said that it would require me to lose a day's salary and asked if I could get compensated. He said, "Oh, you don't want to do that."

"Why not?"

"Because it would come out of my fee, and I'll just have add it to your patient's bill from me, so you'd really be taking it out of her pocket, and you know she doesn't have much." That logic certainly didn't apply to lawyers or the lawyer's fees because my patient told me he expected not only payment in full, but payment in advance and at the rate of $300/hour. No *pro bono* here on his part, only on her doctor's part.

This was my first, and I might say only, experience in a courtroom, for which I thank God daily. Luckily her case was the first one so it didn't take all day. When I was called to testify, they gave me the oath. "Do you swear to tell the truth, the whole truth, and nothing but the truth, so help you God?" Now at this time in our history, there was the beginning of a great clamor to remove "God" from everything. They were taking down any posting of the 10 Commandments, protests over our motto, "In God We Trust," prohibiting high school students from praying before or after football games, and even censoring Valedictorian speeches to make sure the graduate didn't happen to thank God for anything. I guess they really wanted to remove God, Himself, from everything but since that couldn't be achieved they settled for removing His name.

So when it came time to swear to tell the truth, I decided, instead of just saying "I do" as would be normal, I would clarify some points about where this court stood. So I said, "Does the taking of this oath mean that the court acknowledges the existence of God?" You would have thought that I set the courtroom on fire. The judge went absolutely ballistic. She actually got up off her chair. I thought she was going to come down to me, have me in cuffs and put me in jail. With fire breathing from her mouth, she directed the court clerk to "administer him the other oath." The second one had the tag line, at the end, "under penalty of perjury" rather than "so help you God." So I avoided a contempt of court charge, gave my testimony and went home. I don't know if my patient ever got what she was looking for but I do know the lawyer got his fee and the courtrooms thereafter were kept God free.

CHAPTER 12

What's the worst thing that could happen?

When it was my turn to be Chief of the Medicine Department, I got to know some of the medical staff secretaries. A lot of pressure was put on them to get paper work done, expedite applications, type up minutes to the meetings and generally kiss the feet of the staff president, who loved having his feet kissed. (What was quite surprising was that he didn't have them give him a massage as well.) At one particularly bad time, I walked into the medical staff office, and found Jane Johnson in tears. She had papers she was working through very meticulously, piled up on her desk. She didn't want to make any mistakes. She was already working 4 nights a week, and taking work home with her, but just wasn't getting them completed. Her home life was suffering, her marriage was breaking, she was becoming a nervous wreck, and she didn't see any end in sight.

I felt that I had to give her the *hakuna matata* philosophy about paper work, which I learned from Dr. Bill, the paperwork wizard. I told Jane that all the years that Dr. Bill had practiced at the hospital and all the years that I had practiced so far, I never heard of a patient dying from a lack of paperwork being filled out.

"Just make sure all the boxes are checked and move on. Half the time it doesn't really make any difference with regard to patient care if some of the boxes are checked correctly, or just checked. So just make sure all the important boxes are checked correctly and you'll be fine. Plus," (and this is what made the difference for her) I said, "Look at it this way, no matter what kind of mistakes you make, nobody dies. The rest of us have to worry about that. You don't. So lighten up, and don't worry about it." And she did, and she got the job done, and no one ever found unchecked or wrongly checked boxes. Later, upon her retirement from her job, she told me how much that "talk" meant to her and how it changed her attitude, and probably saved her marriage.

A Special Kind of Crazy

After my stint as Chief of Medicine, I was asked to be on the Board of Directors of the Connecticut Academy of Family Physicians. This would never have happened in real life because this was a pretty closed group. Not as bad as the Skull and Bones or membership for the Augusta National Golf Course, but you did need to know someone, who was already on the board, and they had to recommend you, and vouch for you. It turned out I showed up on their radar through the Tar Wars program, which was developed and sponsored by the American Academy of Family Physicians. It seemed that I was the only family doc, in the entire state, who was actually doing these presentations. The national guys wanted to know from the state guys, who was this doc who was sending posters in from his state for the national poster contest. They didn't want any Lone Rangers or wild cowboys who were unsupervised. They had never heard of me, but made it a point to find out who I was. So they contacted me, and asked if I would like to be on the board, and, oh, by the way, be the state coordinator of the Tar Wars program. I thought, "Sure. I guess I can coordinate myself pretty well." So I agreed to be on the board.

But I was not satisfied with just trying to recruit and coordinate the Tar Wars programs. I wanted this group to actually do something helpful for the family docs in our state. So I spoke out about addressing the skyrocketing malpractice insurance costs, as well as, the increasing governmental and insurances' financial control over our practices. Initially, it seemed I struck a chord with the others on the board, because they moved me up the chairs, and eventually elected me President. At that point I wanted to move in a certain direction, and everyone else thought I had gone off the rails.

I was requested to testify before the state assembly to lobby for lower malpractice premiums. In order to testify it was required to be at the statehouse at 8:30 AM on the morning one was scheduled to testify, even though one could be called anytime between 10 AM and 4 PM, with no indication as to when, or not called at all. There were no guarantees. All depended on how "busy" they were. Secondly, when one is called to testify before a particular committee, such as I was, one would reasonably expect the committee to be present to hear the testimony. We've all seen those scenes on TV or movies where the Senate committee was all lined up, and the witness, like Don Corleone, was sitting facing them, making his statement, answering questions or taking the Fifth Amendment to not incriminate himself. That did not happen. Out of about 17 representatives on this insurance commission, anywhere from 3 to 4 were present at any one time. Some would even get up in the middle of a testimony and leave. Others would show up for a few minutes and leave again. Not even the Chairman of the committee was there the whole time. The disinterest in hearing the pro and con arguments was clearly overwhelming.

That experience unlocked the mystery of how our representatives vote. It has nothing to do with listening to their constituents, knowing the facts, or even being interested in knowing the facts, and supporting the best position. They already knew how they were going to vote. They had their minds made up before the hearings even started, most likely because they had all been bought and paid for by the lobbyists, and told which position to take.

Malpractice premiums stabilized only when family docs gave up OB and other "high risk" procedures, even though they were trained to do them, and had no suits or claims. But the rest of the insurance industry began to chime in on how expensive these doctors were for them. They just couldn't pay all these claims. (Good grief. Cry me a river. They were all making a fortune, and paying their CEO's millions, but they couldn't afford to cover their doctors?)

It was also at that time that insurance and governmental regulations and paperwork were becoming overwhelming. Every small office needed at least 2-3 full time employees just to deal with insurance and government issues—pre-authorizations, denial of payment, rebilling with the "correct code" or submitting extra explanations of procedures and benefits, resubmissions of "lost claims"—all of which led said employees to spend hours on the telephone on hold trying to get through to the right department. Once connected to the knowledgeable person, they would not tell you what the problem or error was with the claim that necessitated a denial of service or payment or both. You had to guess what it might be. It was costing us a lot of money and wasting a lot of time. That is, of course, if you didn't mysteriously get disconnected while waiting on hold.

This is when I came to the conclusion that no one in government or in the insurance industry was interested in making our jobs easier or better, for either the doctors or their patients. So with the smell of rotten fish still on me, I began to lobby the board hard to take matters into their own hands and control their own destiny. My suggestion was that as a group, we drop all insurance, and take care of our patients without worrying about what the insurance will cover, or how much they would be reimbursed. (You have to understand, this was the equivalent of throwing tea in Boston harbor. It was a declaration of independence from all the industries that controlled us.) That's when I got the "We can't do that" response. "Why not?" "Because we won't get paid." "Correct. You will have to get paid by your patients, and you will have to charge less, but you will no longer be a high priced prostitute for those trying to control the medical practices in our country."

As you can guess, that comment did not go over well. They all saw themselves as altruistic, self-sacrificing, hard-working servants for a great cause. And they were. But they were also selling their services to the highest bidder. The doctors were providing a service for one group of people (their patients), but expecting another group (the insurance companies) to pay for the services rendered to the first group. The second group did not care about the provision or the quality of the service to the first group, only how much it cost. And it was they who set the price, not the service provider or the service receiver (as it is in any other free transaction between people). Since it is the second group that determines the price, the doctors are then forced to do the will and pleasure of this second group (third party payers), at times to the detriment of the first group (the patients). (He who pays the piper calls the tune that everyone will dance to.) At least a prostitute gets to set her own price. The doctors weren't even at that level. We were already no longer called "doctors." We were addressed now as "medical providers," "health care providers" or "primary care providers." We were stripped of our professionalism and professional title. Why would we put up with that? Lawyers get paid by the minute for keeping people out of jail and we couldn't even get paid a living wage for keeping people out of the cemetery.

What I didn't realize at the time, but which became more evident as time passed, was that the insurance companies and the government were colluding in this matter. The government wanted to control the cost of Medicare and government supplied health insurances. The government also wanted to "save the Social Security system from bankruptcy." What better way to do this than to have people die sooner so as to not be able to collect their Social Security checks? (Of course they never considered not putting any and all who had a drug addiction, alcoholism, ADD, HIV or any and all other "disabilities" on the Social Security system, which was originally meant for those over 65.) This all came to light when Obamacare was passed and they had "panels" to determine who was eligible for care—care not based on efficacy, appropriateness or need, but rather on the "cost to society to keep this person alive." Even AARP, who supposedly represented the retired and elderly, endorsed this plan.

One of the big initiatives while I was on the FP board was the institution of electronic medical records. Some docs were really on board with it, and others were saying, "I don't know if this is a step forward or backward." One member was all gung ho and instituted an electronic medical record system in his office, with the help, and financial backing of one of the electronic medical record systems companies. He then made a presentation about how it went, and especially all the advantages of having an electronic system. It was just great if you wanted to find out Mrs. X's blood sugar report from 1947, and it was the cat's meow when it came to printing out prescriptions, or better yet, faxing them directly to the pharmacy. However, someone had to enter all the data from the paper charts. This could be done by hiring an agency to do this, or it could be done by the doctor and his staff on nights, weekends and holidays when they didn't have to take care of actual real time patients. Of course they could also enter the data at the patient's regular appointment, but that would require a 45 min to an hour appointment, while they got used to the system, and got the information transferred.

The transition could take up to 2 years, although one could be "up and running" in as little as 6-9 months, but until then they'd have to see less than half the number of patients they normally see, while they were getting "up and running." Oh, the best part, without the financial incentives from the company, it would have cost him $50,000/month in lost revenue to institute this, and that didn't include updates and user fees. And what were the "good" points? The insurance companies were offering "incentives" in the form of payment for those who got a medical record system. If you had an electronic record, the insurance company would pay a premium for an office visit. This was supposed to make up for the fall off in income. One thing that was very suspicious was that the insurance companies, the federal government, and the national medical organizations were all singing the same song and pushing hard for these records. Why? Well everyone found out later.

Being the President of state FP board got me a ticket to go to the National American Academy meetings. This is where the disillusionment with the whole political aspect of medicine really came to the forefront. I thought, "It is probably all my fault. I expected that the Academy cared about the family docs out in the country, who were working, and trying to care for their patients as best as they could." I saw the AAFP as an advocate for those docs. Little did I know that the foxes were already in this hen house.

All the resolutions passed at these meetings had to do with social advocacy and none with the well-being of the family docs in the field. They were more interested in having abortions available, alternative lifestyles advanced and advocated, children being allowed to be adopted by gay couples, and catering to women, minorities, foreign-born and alternative living life style advocacy groups than they were in the docs out in the country trying to scratch out a living in the midst of increasing governmental and insurance regulations. With regard to government mandates, they were complicit with and in favor of them. With regard to progressive social agendas, they were advocates. With regard to the crushing requirements placed on doctors and their practices, they rolled over and played dead.

There is nothing worse than realizing that someone, who you counted on to be your advocate and ally, betrays you, and gives you up to the enemy. (Perhaps a little melodramatic but true nonetheless). What do you do when your lawyer decides you have to plead guilty to charges you did not commit, and if you don't, he's off the case? It was then I realized: "They no longer represent me. I have to resign."

CHAPTER 13

Clara

Another patient who came in for a check-up one summer day was an elderly lady, Clara. She always came to the office with Ralph, her husband. She was a nervous wreck and worried about everything. Clara was brought up in Sarasota, Florida. She was raised in a good home as a strict Southern Baptist but, for some inexplicable reason, always had a rebellious spirit. Her mother and father tried to keep control over her, but Clara just wouldn't have it. She was always attracted to the "bad boys" in her town, and her parents were always sure she would wind up pregnant. Now Sarasota also happened to be the winter home of the circus and Ralph was traveling with the circus as a tattoo artist. To a young girl, this looked like a life of excitement and adventure, and Ralph was the ultimate bad boy covered in tattoos. So in 1921, in her 18th year, when the circus pulled out of town, Clara went with it. She travelled all over the country and worked for the circus at odd jobs. There was a "painted lady" who was also traveling with the circus at the same time. This tattooed lady was part of the side show, and made extra money because of her tattoos. Clara was thinking maybe she could do the same, until the painted lady asserted her place in that role by threatening to kill Clara if she took her place. Clara was told in no uncertain terms that there was only room for one tattooed lady.

She got very involved with Ralph, who had been involved with the painted lady previously - probably another reason the painted lady disliked Clara so much. Ralph practiced his craft on Clara to the point that there was hardly a place, except for her face, that did not have a tattoo. When I asked her if she would get the same tattoos again, if she had to do it over, she told me, "Hell, no. I wouldn't get any of them. They look hideous." And then would cast a withering glance at her husband.

I guess once again proving that some of the wild oats that are sown while young, grow up to be thorns and thistles that are not quite as pleasing when we are older.

Jerry and Martha

Jerry and Martha were neighbors of ours. Jerry was a retired fireman from NY City and Martha was his wife of many years. Jerry met her while in the army, when he was stationed in Georgia at Fort Benning. Martha was working on the base as a secretary. After a whirlwind romance, they wanted to get married. Martha's father was not happy with this marriage and refused to attend the wedding. He just could not cotton to this Yankee marrying his daughter, especially a Catholic Yankee. "That's the worst kind you know."

In spite of the opposition from her father, Martha got married to Jerry in the rectory of Our Lady of the Confederacy, because as a non-Catholic, Martha was not allowed to darken the doors of the Catholic Church to be married. Afterward they moved to N.Y. where Jerry got a job as a fireman and raised 5 daughters with Martha. After retiring from the fire department, they moved up to our town to be near their daughter, whose husband had a job as supervisor in one of the mills.

Jerry had sustained a serious injury one day while fighting a fire. He fell down some rotten burned out stairs and hurt his back. It hurt him every day afterward but he didn't want to quit the job or go on disability. He would medicate it the best way he could.

Every afternoon around 4, Jerry would say to Martha, "Martha, I'll take a Manhattan."

"It's not even 5 o'clock yet," Martha would always answer.

"Oh, OK. We can wait."

"Well, it's 5 o'clock somewhere," Martha would say as she relented, and would give him a full bodied Manhattan.

So every afternoon, Jerry and Martha would go through this routine and have a Manhattan each. Then another. And then a third. After three, they'd stop counting. What Jerry didn't know was that Martha was starting way ahead of him, and had 3 Manhattans down already when he asked for his first one. I was afraid that someday someone would find them passed out, face down in their oatmeal.

But that never happened. What did happen was one day Martha called for me to come over quickly. When I got there, I found Jerry on the floor.

"Did he fall?"

"Not actually," said Martha.

"Did he pass out?" guessing again.

"Not actually," Martha said again.

"Well, what did happen, actually?"

"Do you think we need to call the ambulance?" Martha asked.

At this point Jerry entered the conversation. "No ambulance. I'll be alright. I just need a little rest."

"Well, I think there are better places to rest than in the middle of the living room floor," I said.

"I'll be alright. I just got a little dizzy when I got up, and got down on the floor and couldn't get back up. My back wouldn't let me."

"How many drinks have you had?"

"I don't know. Four, maybe five. What difference does that make?"

I looked at Martha who nodded her head in agreement.

Since he moved to town the episodes of severe back pain were getting worse. He continued self-medicating himself with escalating doses of Manhattans, maybe to remind himself where this accident took place.

There were times Jerry was totally disabled with this, to the point of being bedridden. Other days were better and he'd be able to work around the house, but he would be in pain every day.

I asked Jerry if he wanted me to make an appointment with a pain specialist for him, and told him I would drive him there myself. He kept refusing until the pain finally got to the point that he gave in to my constant harassment.

The day of the appointment, we gathered all of Jerry's X-Rays, MRI's and CT Scans to bring along with us. The MRI showed a ruptured disc that was said to be inoperable. I initially thought maybe some epidural injections might help.

We went in to see Dr. Jenkins, a spine specialist. Dr. Jenkins looked over the previous studies, examined Jerry, and said he could see where he could have some pain. The day we went up there, Jerry was having one of his better days, but Dr. Jenkins gave him an epidural and told him to come back in 4-6 weeks for a recheck.

After they got home, Martha and Jack noticed that Jerry's pain was much worse. He could hardly move most of the time. His daily Manhattans started about 2 PM and stopped after about 10 drinks. And Martha would match him drink for drink. This was not a good situation, I said to myself, and also to Jerry and Martha's daughters, Jennifer and Judy. Telling the daughters did not make me a friend to Jerry or Martha. He didn't want his daughters to know his business because they had no business in his affairs.

But as it turned out, his daughters were essential to his care. They came over every afternoon to look in on him. Martha, after about 7

Manhattans, would usually fall asleep in her recliner and Jerry would be writhing with the pain he denied he had.

When it came time for Jerry's follow up visit, Jerry, Martha and Jennifer now all went with him. Jerry made it clear that he didn't want anyone coming into the doctor's office with him. This was his visit, and he wanted it to be in private.

When they arrived, Jerry was so incapacitated that he couldn't get out of the car without help, and needed a wheelchair to get into the office. "Good," Jennifer thought. "This doctor will finally see him at his worst, and maybe discover something that may have been missed the first visit."

Jerry was taken into the office by himself. When he came out, he looked good until he got outside the waiting room door, when he practically collapsed to the ground. All drove back disappointed. They all asked Jerry what the doctor said. "Nothing. He said I'm doing good." "How could you be doing good when you can hardly walk?" "I'm fine." This conversation played over and over on the way back home.

Another follow up in 6 weeks. The same scenario, but this time Jennifer insisted on going in to see what the doctor actually said. Jerry's name was called, and Jennifer and Jerry went into the exam room. The conversation went like this:

Doctor: Well how have you been doing since our last visit?

Jerry: I've been doing good. The pain is much better.

Jennifer: You've got to be kidding. The pain has been excruciating and you've been practically bedridden. How can you tell him you've been doing good?

Jerry: Don't pay any attention to her. She doesn't know what she's talking about. I'm doing fine.

Doctor: Well let me see how you can move and bend.

With that Jerry gets up out of the chair and practically does pirouettes. Jennifer was flabbergasted.

Doctor: Well it looks like you're just about back to normal. You won't need any more follow up appointments.

As they walked out of the exam room, again Jerry's knees buckled, and they had to carry him back to his car.

After they got home Jennifer related to me what had happened in the office. I was incredulous. "Jerry, do you know how many calls and strings I had to pull to get you in to see this guy, and you lie to him about how you're doing?"

"He said I'm doing good, and he's the doctor, so he should know. Don't worry about me."

I was practically apoplectic. His daughters were demoralized to the point that they were making novenas to St. Ann for the "good Lord to take him home and relieve him of his suffering."

Eventually the "good Lord" answered the girls' prayers, but not until they were practically tearing out their hair trying to make him comfortable. It seemed the only place he was comfortable was in that spine doctor's examining room. No one could understand it.

J.L.

J.L. was a 50's yr. old lady who worked in a mill and whose husband did the same. She lived a modest life, but always seemed to have money problems. Some of these stemmed from the fact that her children would "borrow" money, and then forget to pay it back, so in essence she was still supporting them, even though they were adults with adult expenses.

One day J came in ecstatic. She had won the lottery. Not the hundreds of millions but about $5 million. After the Feds took their piece she still had plenty to spend—and she did. She bought new cars, a house and gifts for family and friends. What could go wrong?

About 6 months later, she came in very depressed saying she had no money. “How could you not have any money? You won the lottery?” She just cried that she was broke. Then she said, “Can you believe they want me to pay taxes on the money I already spent? I thought the money was mine.” (The state wanted taxes and the feds wanted some sort of adjustment tax from her.) “So just pay them,” I suggested. “I can’t. I spent it all. I don’t have any money to pay the taxes.” I don’t know how she worked things out with the IRS, but she never hit the lottery again, or had any extra money again, and went back on welfare, and pretty much died broke. The lottery advertising slogan was “If you don’t play, you can’t win.” But for J.L., she played, she supposedly won, but in the end still lost.

Margaret

I met Chuck and Margaret when they moved to the area when Chuck retired. They had raised 2 children and perhaps 60 foster children in their younger days. They moved back to the family house. The house was a large colonial and in their family since the Revolutionary War. It was *the* family heirloom.

Their own children were wealthy high rollers living in New York, and they rarely saw them. When Chuck died suddenly, Margaret basically lived in 2 rooms on the first floor of the house. She couldn’t afford to heat the rest of the house in the winter, and it was easier to keep 2 or 3 rooms cool with a window air-conditioner.

As Margaret aged she found it more difficult to get around. Neighbors and friends would pitch in to take her shopping, to church and to the cemetery to visit Chuck’s grave. She would come into the office and talk about her decreasing financial status, wondering how she was going to keep her house and pay the expenses. I suggested she may want to sell the house, as it was too big and costing her more than she could afford. That she said she would never do.

It was about this time when her son's daughter decided to go to University in Connecticut at Storrs. Her son would come and see her once or twice a year when he either picked up or dropped off his daughter at school. It was during one of these visits when she decided that she would give the house to her son and then go on government assistance. Not long after that decision, her son decided she should go into a nursing home and have the State of Connecticut pay for all his mother's expenses.

I asked her how she felt about this arrangement and she was overjoyed. Her son would get the house, it would stay in the family, and her expenses would all be paid for. She couldn't ask for more. From the time she went into the nursing home until her death, her son was just too busy to visit her. Mother's day and holidays would all pass without a visit. My wife would take her to put flowers on Chuck's grave every Memorial Day, but her son, daughter or grandchildren never came to see her.

About a week after Margaret died, her house, her pride and joy, her heirloom to bequeath to her family so they could live there, went up for sale. Her son had figured out a way to not have to care for or pay for care for his mother and also make a profit in the end. It was sad to see. The lesson was clear. Don't expect the next generation to value the same things you do.

Eeyore

Eeyore was what I called him. He was an elderly guy who had a lot of minor things wrong. Now you have to understand the categories of illness for doctors. There's critical which generally lead to death. There's serious which can be life threatening if not taken care of. There's minor treatable which do not interfere with one's daily life. And finally minor untreatable, which do interfere with activities of daily living to some degree. Eeyore's was the last type. When he would come in he would sound just like the Winnie the Pooh character. Life was bad, nothing went right, nothing was going well, etc. It just went on and on. Nothing tasted good, he couldn't hear as well as he used to, he'd have to get up from bed at night to use the bathroom, then had trouble getting back to sleep, reading would make him tired, he had to sit down when dressing or he'd lose his balance.... After 10 minutes with him most people wanted to go out and shoot themselves, he got them so depressed. Luckily he had a wife, or I should say a sainted wife, who not only doted on him and waited on him hand and foot, but was able to put up with his chronic complaining.

Both his wife and I would try to get him to concentrate on all the things he could do and all the abilities he did have at 80 years old. I was sure that if he could just concentrate and focus on all the things he was able to do, his life would be much more pleasurable, but he would have none of it. His wife said that when he finally died, she was going to put on his grave stone, "See I told you I was sick."

Disability can be Disabling

Len was a guy in his early 40's who hurt his back. He came to see me complaining that he couldn't do any kind of meaningful work and just had to get on disability. He couldn't sit, stand, or walk for more than 10 minutes without getting excruciating back pain. He would come in with a different story and different symptoms each visit. I referred him to all sorts of back pain specialists but all failed to help him in the slightest. Finally, after about a year and a half of this, I asked him point blank, "If I could cure you of your back pain, would you want me to?" He looked at me with a stunned look of panic and said, "Would that mean I'd have to go to work? I can't go to work. I wouldn't be able to find a job. Who'd hire me with my history? I can't lose my disability."

So the answer was "No." He was too comfortable with his disability to want to be cured.

The Joy of Delivering Babies

There are certain delivery experiences that are seared in your mind forever. Here are some of mine.

While in labor a young lady, who was accompanied by her mother, was coming along nicely, so the nurse and I expected a fairly uneventful delivery. The nurse knew me and my twisted sense of humor, and would sometimes say things that I thought would be humorous, while no one else did. After I delivered the baby boy, I checked the mom as I prepared to deliver the placenta, and I felt another head. I said, "Wait, I think there's another baby in here." (This was way before ultrasounds, which today would find that out before the delivery.) "Don't even joke about that," the young mom said. "What do you think that's funny? That's not funny," her mother added. "Don't be fooling around," the nurse scolded. I told them I was not joking; I was serious. Then I delivered the baby brother twin—my first set of twins. Surprise.

Another incident was when I examined my patient, who came into the labor room in labor, and found out that the baby was in a breach position (head up instead of head down). When that happened, you had 3 choices: 1- do a C-Section, 2- call an obstetrician and they may deliver it as a breach delivery or 3- turn the baby so it delivers head down. Since I didn't want to put the patient through a C-Section or put the baby through the trauma of a breach delivery, I elected # 3. I turned the baby and delivered it normally, and everything turned out fine. However, when the case was reviewed at the OB Department meeting, I was reprimanded and told I wasn't an obstetrician, so I shouldn't perform or know how to perform that procedure, because that's not how it's done here. I told them we did it all the time in my residency training; plus, the baby turned out fine. Then they moved on to another topic. But they had to put me in my place, which, of course, was below them.

Carol had just moved into town and came to see me for her 3rd pregnancy. She was the most kind, most considerate and most generous person I have ever had the pleasure to take care of. Her due date was around Christmas, and we took bets on whether we would be together on Christmas day. As it happened, Christmas morning, she calls me very apologetic. She was sooo sorry, but she was in labor. We both made our way into the hospital, and she rapidly delivered her Christmas baby boy. Throughout the labor and delivery, she kept apologizing for getting me out on Christmas morning to do this, and keeping me from my family. She would not accept that I loved being there with her, and didn't mind in the least. But she was the most considerate patient I ever had. She even had the baby early enough so that I could be home to watch the kids open their presents. I told her that she was the patient by which all other patients will be measured up against. And everyone else lost.

Kurt and Greta were trying to have a baby for some time, so when she finally became pregnant, they were ecstatic. That didn't wear off through the entire pregnancy. Finally they called in the wee hours of the morning saying that Greta was in labor. I made my way to hospital before dawn's early light and delivered a baby boy. That's when Kurt began the Paul Revere routine right there in the delivery room. He just had to call everyone he knew to tell them. The first number he dialed was my phone number. When my sleeping wife answered the phone he realized that he dialed the wrong number, but he didn't miss a beat. He went on to tell her he had a boy, the weight and length. My wife congratulated them, and asked if I'd be home soon, and should she make breakfast. He said, "No, he'll be awhile, but I'll be over in a half hour because I'm hungry." Amazing how becoming a father for the first time can give you an appetite.

Anita

Anita was very anxious, very dependent and insistent on my being there for her whenever and wherever she needed me. One unfortunate time, Anita had to be admitted to the hospital the day before I had to go to my week of National Guard duty in Washington, DC. She was crying and carrying on telling me I couldn't go, and leave her at such a time when she needed me. She told me to tell them I couldn't go, and she tried to call the governor, the president and anyone else she could think of. But since neither the governor nor the President answered her calls, in the end I went to the Pentagon, and she got better. But she never let me forget my abandonment of her in her "greatest time of need."

Claudia

Claudia was a lady, who I initially met while taking care of her mother and father. We hit it off well, and had a very enjoyable time when she and her family came to the office. One time when Claudia was in the office, she showed me a picture of some old folks in a local nursing home "celebrating the 4th of July." They were pictured with ridiculous looking hats on, holding flags and having dazed and confused looks on their faces. She instructed me that should she ever end up in one of "those places," I was to never allow this kind of picture to be taken of her. If I did she'd never forgive me, and come back and haunt me. Every visit after that one, I would tell her how I was going to dress her up for her picture, and she would say, "You better not or else."

When she moved to a retirement community, she related that she would sit outside of her apartment, and other women would come up to talk to her. I said that was nice of them to make you feel welcomed. "Feel welcomed nothing," she said. "They're just busybodies who want to know my business. I tell them to get lost. All they do is gossip." I guess one might say she wasn't receptive to their overtures.

Her son, Jack, loved the outdoors, and was a surveyor. Jack would come in a few times a year to test my dermatology knowledge and skills. He'd have rashes, poison ivy, sumac, oak, bites from all kinds of creatures, Lyme Disease and anything else you could get. I always recommended he get a desk job. He said if he did that, I'd never get to treat these skin problems, so he was just helping with my education. And he probably did.

CHAPTER 14

Who would believe?

As the time passed it brought with it new winds of change. Beliefs that were once thought foundational were now being challenged. Issues came up that I never thought would come up nor be so jolting to the order of things.

One of the big campaigns during this time was to have abortions available at the hospital. The big problem was that all the obstetricians were Roman Catholic, and wouldn't do them. The solution: bring in Planned Parenthood, and they would supply docs who had no objections or scruples of conscious, to do the abortions for them. This was presented in such glowing terms, it almost had the effect of an intoxicating brew—"This is a needed service for the poor and disadvantaged. These women are getting abortions out of town and are made to drive so far away (poor things) while we could supply the service for them right here." (Supply them? Like they were getting office supplies?) And, most persuasive, from the hospital board's point of view: "The hospital will benefit very well financially from these procedures. It will practically print money." (Oh, well, why wasn't that said in the first place? That just seals the deal.) The only ones who were objecting and pushing back against the board, against this proposition, were the obstetricians, but that was enough to stall it, until others could be rallied—nurses, patients and some other docs.

The local Roman Catholic Church, which always opposed abortion, and to which many of the town folks belonged, was approached to bring their influence to bear on the issue. Father Maurice said this was too political, and that it was a decision for the bishop to make.

When the bishop's office was contacted, he said that this is a dilemma that the laity should get involved in, sort out and solve. When asked if he would at least write a letter, and have it read on Sunday, alerting the "laity" of the move to do abortions at the local hospital, he said, "No," he couldn't do that. "Too controversial and not something the clergy should get involved with." (Since when did the Catholic Church consider opposing abortions controversial? You'd think he was up for election and running for cardinal or something, and didn't want to offend anyone.)

During this time 2 obstetricians died of mysterious illnesses, and a third left to join the Navy (said he was tired of having to pay a food taster to make sure he also wasn't going to be found dead of "natural causes"). The controversy died when a couple of new obstetricians who didn't have the same moral scruples about doing abortions came on staff.

A couple of years following the abortion issue, another proposal that came before the board was the introduction of alternative medicine practices at the hospital. A group of nurses were pushing hard to be able to perform certain "non-harmful, but potentially very healing" procedures on the patients. The main ones were therapeutic touch and Reiki.

Therapeutic touch was like magic performed by the shamans of the past. Even though it was called therapeutic *touch,* no touching was ever done. They just hovered their hands over the patient. This was supposed to rearrange, and straighten out their energy fields thus making them feel better. (Now, most docs have no problem with you giving them a shot for pain, or doing surgery on them, but don't mess with their energy fields. They need all the energy they can get and can't afford some amateur playing around with them or short circuiting them by mistake.) The real issue with this therapeutic modality was there was no scientific evidence that energy fields even existed, let alone that they could be the cause of illness, or that they could be manipulated by hands held over someone, or that this was helpful to anyone. (The question was: Was the hospital a facility that treated people according to the best scientific evidence available or by magic? Now lest you think this was a no brainer, the magic voting folks had a fairly large contingent. Again the hospital board wanted to be open and affirming of all types of treatments, even bogus ones, especially if there was money to be made.)

The other therapeutic modality was Reiki. This practice also corrected your energy fields, but this one with the aid and assistance of a spirit guide. (Now, anything that calls down spirits of unknown reputation, is not something some of the medical staff wanted to foster on unwary patients. Also understand that at this time, not even the chaplains were allowed to call on Jesus Christ to heal patients, but unknown spirits were deemed to pass the test of "authentic." Go figure.)

The odd thing about this whole controversy was the involvement of the minister of the Congregational Church. It seemed that his son had gone away to study with some yogi, and learned Eastern religion and transcendental meditation, and practiced some of these magical arts. It wasn't that he was behind the whole movement, but he certainly galvanized enough support for it from his congregation that it made it a going concern.

This same minister actually had come into my office one day with a TIME magazine. The cover was an Easter theme, with something about "Did Jesus really rise from the dead?" At the end of the visit, he shows me the cover and says, "Do you believe that Christ rose from the dead?" I, thinking that I was on fairly solid ground speaking to a pastor, said I did. To which this minister said, "I don't believe He rose bodily. I think it was a spiritual thing." "Oh, good, I'm glad to know that. Now I want you to continue on the same blood pressure meds. Do you need any prescriptions?"

Oh, no. It wasn't going to be that easy. He had to have me defend my belief in the bodily resurrection of Christ, and had to thrust, parry and riposte with him for 45 minutes before he was convinced that I was totally ignorant of higher Biblical criticism and the more enlightened views.

On another occasion, he asked me if I believed the book of Genesis was true. Again I said, for the most part, yes. "You mean to tell me you believe in this Adam and Eve stuff. What about evolution? You're a man of science. How can you believe that ####?" That time he and I went around the idea of what it means for man to be created in God's image, original sin and the fall of mankind, all of which he was not buying. Again it was 45 minutes before we could resolve this issue to his satisfaction that I was a total idiot, when it came to theology.

So when I found out that this man's son belonged to an ashram, and was a yogi, and both he and his wife thought that these Eastern religious ideas were wonderful, it all came together for me. If I had known I was arguing with someone who didn't believe in Christianity, it might have saved me a lot of time and effort. I was under the false impression that we would actually find some area of agreement.

With enough physician opposition, the proposal for "energy therapy" failed that time around. The questions that swirled: "What's next, hospital privileges for witch doctors? What department should we put them in? Oh, I guess we could lump them together with the voodoo practitioners, soothsayers, and magicians, who will also be applying for privileges." At that time no one would have imagined that someday the proposal would succeed. They really created a Dept. of Magic Arts or Alternative Medicine, as it is now labeled as its official title.

When Medicine Ceased to be Medical

One of the most frustrating aspects to practicing medicine in the hospital, was that it was becoming more of a business than a caring facility. The policies were being dictated by lawyers, not by physicians. On entering the hospital as a patient, one was presented 17 pages of disclaimers and warnings, notifying them that they are taking all risks and assuming all responsibility if anything goes wrong, so don't blame us because we told you so.

Before admission, patients are required to determine just how much medical care they want to receive. Do they want to be resuscitated if their heart stops, do they want to be cremated or buried, and what do they want written on their grave stone. ("But I just cut my hand and need some stitches." "Doesn't matter. It's required by our attorneys.")

Along with their advanced directives, they are required to submit their obituary, and in which papers they would want it published, with required statements included that would exonerate the hospital of any and all responsibility of whatever were to happen. (This is an exaggeration to be sure, but not by much.)

Before procedures, patients are now given verbal warnings of all the possible side effects—all side effects, no matter how unlikely. I personally liked the one that said you could get killed by a meteor if it struck the hospital during your stay, and the hospital was not responsible for any of your injuries. It's like listening to the fine print on a prescription print out being read to you twice as fast as you could actually listen. After a while the patient zones out and stops hearing anything, thus missing the really important and likely side effects that actually could happen. They all agree to anything, just to make the nurse stop describing everything to them. The most amusing statement made during this exchange is, that after hearing all this, the patient is asked, "Do you have any questions?" (Any questions? Yeah I've got a lot of questions. But I don't know if I should ask about the possibility of getting ingrown toenails from this procedure or the possibility of developing an allergy to talcum powder.)

Becoming a business entity now requires the hospital to send out surveys to make sure the patient had a pleasant stay. Now who wouldn't want to receive twelve 25 page surveys from the hospital administrator, the head of the nursing department, the anesthesiologist, the IV nurse, the surgeon, the internist, the hospitalist, the pharmacist, the scrub nurse, the circulating nurse, the dietary department and the housekeeping person that cleaned your room.

Where do all these surveys go, you might ask. They all go to the public relations department who cull them for key phrases they can use in their advertising brochures. Phrases like, "better than being at a 5 star resort," "fine dining at its best," "best surgeon I ever had, didn't even leave a scar," "nurse treated me nicer than my own mother," and "would highly recommend this hospital to all my friends." Of course statements like "I wouldn't send my dog to that guy," "rat infested," "food made me vomit," and "waited 14 hours for the nurse to answer my call light" didn't make it into the brochures.

When Wisdom Is More Precious Than Gold

It was a typical day for me until Don Wilson, the pastor of the Evangelical Church came in to tell me that I will soon find out that he would be leaving town. He and I had gotten to know one another well, and always had a theological discussion during his visits. I always thought him to be caring, personable and very knowledgeable of the Bible, and a good pastor. One could see why the Evangelical Church was growing. People liked him. He had a very gentle way about him.

When I asked why he was leaving, and where was he going, he said that the church was firing him. He was summarily dismissed by some leadership elders, who told him to immediately clean out his desk, took his keys and escorted him out of the church. Not quite a perp walk to the police station, but very close. Now how often does a church fire a successful pastor? Almost never except for a severe breach of conduct. When asked why, Don said he would rather not talk about it. He felt it was a minor molehill that was being made into Mount Everest.

At the church's congregational meeting, which was called into emergency session, they were all told that Pastor Wilson would be leaving because of a "serious matter." The lead elder had even called in an official of the denomination to oversee this meeting and support the elder's decision. What was very suspect in the whole proceedings, was that this very same elder, had performed the same service at the previous church he was in. He appeared to be a professional pastor assassin.

So when the congregation was assembled, they were told "it was a serious sin." But they wouldn't say what it was in order to "protect this pastor's reputation." Now it appeared to all gathered that his reputation was pretty well shot already. In fact the entire town knew about the happenings at the Evangelical Church. When asked if it was a criminal act, stealing, child molestation, embezzlement of funds or anything that he was apt to be arrested for, they said, "Oh, no, nothing as serious as that."

When questioned whether it was alcoholism, drug use, adultery or teaching heresy, they said, "Oh, no, nothing that bad."

"So is there no treatment, rehabilitation, repentance, forgiveness and restoration possible before taking the step to fire him?" "No, the decision has been made. And unless he further humbles himself by confessing his sin in front of everyone, and begs their forgiveness, there is nothing further to be done." It seemed to most that being publicly fired and accused of terrible sin was humiliation enough, thus opening up a rift in the congregation.

I later found out that the "serious, unforgivable problem" was that Don had clicked a link on his computer which took him to a pornographic webpage. He maintained that it was by mistake, but no one was giving him the benefit of the doubt.

But even the worst of stories has an upside. Don and his family went to Colorado. He became a delivery man for Coors Beer and lived happily ever after.

On the other hand, the Evangelical Church split into the pro-pastor and the anti-pastor factions. The pro-pastor group decided they could not stay in a church that treated their pastor so shabbily, and the other churches in the area gained new members. So it's an ill wind that blows no one any good. But it does show that forgiveness is not in our DNA, even in those who had themselves been forgiven. And wisdom requires a daily application of when to forgive and when to ask for forgiveness.

Strange Times

Speaking of pastors, one person I was never able to engage in conversation was Pastor Darrell Smith. Darrell was the pastor of the Methodist Church in town. He was married and had 2 children, two boys. At the time I was seeing him, his boys were 14 and 12. His wife, Pamela, worked as a social worker to supplement their income. They appeared to be just perfect for pastoring the Methodist Church.

Darrell worked out at the gym and was a physical fitness enthusiast. Up at 5 AM running 5-10 miles, then working out at least 5 days a week. His wife was also very health conscience. She was a strict vegetarian and she kept him on a vegetarian diet as well. She was involved with a woman's workout group in the mornings and then off to work. Interestingly their boys were not as much into physical activity as their parents. Tom, the oldest, was into being creative. He was into drawing and art, and devoured books. Lee, the youngest, was a computer player. When given the choice of what to do, he chose to play some computer game. Neither played sports.

When Darrell came into the office he would never want to talk about how his family was, nor the stress he may have been feeling from his job, nor even theology, like the other ministers would. He would always rebuke me for asking. "I'm here for __________ (fill in the blank), not to talk about anything else." Reluctantly he talked about his exercise program, but that was because he saw that as a health concern, and therefore appropriate to discuss. The good thing about his attitude was that it made for very short visits. The bad thing was I never got to know him as a person, nor as a patient who was made up of more than a physical body.

One day, much to the surprise of everyone, Pastor Darrell Smith submitted his resignation, effective immediately, and moved to Arizona. Now almost everyone, who lived in the north, could understand a move to Arizona. But they did not understand the rest of it. His wife told her friends that she was taking a job in Boston, and her kids would be living with her.

It was only much later that word came about that he had decided to leave his family, and to marry another guy, who he had met at the gym. Even for an open and affirming community, that was a lot to process. They could understand wanting to marry another man, but they were all in a flutter over the fact that he would leave his kids. And why go to Arizona? You could do that right here at home. There were just too many unanswered questions for the town's folks.

What really fed the gossip mill, which was verified by Facebook posts, was that Pamela didn't go to Boston like she said. She went to Tucson. Why would she lie to everyone, people wanted to know. And Tucson was the same city that Darrell told his elders he was going to. Now that information was just too much for Mrs. O'Brien. She was the FBI class investigator in town. She knew more about everyone in town than J. Edgar Hoover ever knew about Al Capone. It wouldn't surprise folks if she had a file on everyone in town, and that upon her death, those files might end up in the wrong hands, and nobody's secrets would be safe.

Mrs. O'Brien made it her business to investigate the "strange case of Darrell Smith." And to no one's surprise found that Darrell, his new husband and who everyone thought was his former wife all lived at the same address. She also discovered that Darrell and Pamela never got divorced. (Access to public records is just amazing today.) So how he was allowed to marry another person was beyond comprehension. She also found out that Darrell and Pamela were married in Las Vegas by an Elvis impersonator in 1974. Now everyone was wondering if they even had a legal wedding. So Mrs. O'Brien after research found they did not have a valid Nevada marriage license on file. Everyone was astonished at how Mrs. O'Brien could find her way around the internet and come up with such delightful morsels for them to chew on.

Years later, Darrell's son Tom, would write a best seller on growing up in a household with 2 fathers and a mother, who made their living by taking young men into their home, and charging them by the hour. For what services the young men were paying just doesn't need to be said. Everyone, who read his book, believed he made the whole story up. Except Mrs. O'Brien, she knew the truth.

Always expect the unexpected I was once told, but you almost never do.

What's happened to the women?

Things were going on in this idyllic town that would have been hard to believe just 10 years before. Another example was on three separate occasions separated by no more than a month, 3 married guys with children came in to see me and were just weeping. They all had the same story. Their wives had left them. Now the story of a wife leaving a husband was not really a new one. But in these instances, they all left their husbands for another woman. The kids were totally confused and just could not understand it, and their dads couldn't explain it because they also didn't understand it. Today this kind of goings on would not be looked at twice, but this was in the day before same sex couples, and homosexual liaisons were kept tightly closeted. But even with today's views, from a naturalistic worldview, I still have difficulty in understanding how the natural affections of one sex for another and the desire for children could be changed to a preference that leads to an evolutionary dead end.

In the end, all the husbands remarried happily. One set of children disowned the mother and would have nothing to do with her, another daughter married another woman, with none of her family condoning it or wishing her luck, and all suffered rejection and a feeling of betrayal, and their scars effected their future relationships. Which leads to the question: When the pursuit of your own happiness leads to the unhappiness of so many others, should your own happiness be pursued at all costs?

CHAPTER 15

When You Own a Business

Glen Skeffington was a very successful, and very busy, business man. He didn't have time to make appointments, and certainly didn't have time to wait in a waiting room for a doctor to see him. He would come in unannounced, wanting to be seen—now. At the same time he'd bring in a box of donuts, coffee, appetizers, calzones, pizza or some other enticements or gifts for the staff. Glen knew the secret key that really opened the doctor's office was the front office staff, and he always got in. I never ever scolded him for messing up my schedule, nor the staff for accepting bribes. In fact I would have liked to encourage everyone to bring in bribes—eggs, chickens, a side of beef, prime rib, beef tenderloin, fresh sweet corn in season or whatever. It was more than the insurance companies were paying us. You would have thought that this type of secret information would be spread around town, and everyone would be doing likewise. But that never happened. Glen knew how to keep a secret and not let any competitors in the door.

Glen had an older brother, Tom, who didn't care to be involved with the business. After high school he went to the Coast Guard Academy. He loved being out on the water sailing the seas. After he finished his obligation to the Coast Guard, he bought a luxury yacht and moved to Miami Beach and rented out his yacht for cruises up and down the inter coastal waterway. In the spring he'd move up to Norfolk, Virginia, and in the summer went to Mystic, Connecticut, and had cruises from there. So no amount of love nor money could coax Tom to get involved in his father's business.

Glenn inherited his business from his father, Charles. Charles worked hard, was a member of the Lutheran Church, and always volunteered to work the Oktoberfest or to do other necessary jobs around the church. He was in town during the famous Blizzard of '55, when they were inundated with 48 inches of snow, a 10 day power outage, and the need to call in the National Guard to help the town get in needed food, water and supplies. Charles was at the forefront in getting this done. He also helped repair the roof on the Grange Hall that had collapsed because of the weight of the snow. Everyone in town loved Charles. They even had a Charles Skeffington Day to honor him in 1978.

Charles started a wooden dowel making factory. He supplied wooden dowels to hundreds of furniture makers, builders, cabinet makers and those who needed wooden rods. It was very successful. He and his wife, Betty, became two of the pillars of the community. His competitiveness was only in the realm of business. He wanted to make the best dowels for the best price. He felt that if you didn't strive for excellence, you would never achieve it. And his business thrived.

Charles had raised Glenn with a bit of an entitlement attitude. Glen never had to really work for anything. Whatever he needed was provided by his father. Glen, unlike his dad, went to a private prep school and then college, played sports and upon marriage was able to afford a house, with Charles giving him a sizable down payment. Glen learned his father's business, and was expected to take it over after his father retired. He had inherited his father outgoing personality, and was liked by everyone who met him. But what Glen did not inherit was the business climate in which his father worked and thrived. When Charles went into business, it was assumed that if you worked hard, and were cautious with your spending, you would succeed. If you weren't succeeding, it was because you weren't working hard enough or wasted money on frivolous things like vacations, second houses, yachts or expensive cars.

By the time Glen took over, it wasn't enough to work hard. Now you were expected to work 'smart," which was another way of saying you needed to "cut deals." If you wanted to sell your dowels, you had to sell your soul as well. You had to bribe the buyer with gifts, money, trips. Glen couldn't believe he had to do business like this, but if he wanted to continue his father's business, he seemed to have no choice. Eventually these "deals" were beginning to eat away at his profits. On top of that, the state kept raising the taxes on his business because as they said, "He had to pay his fair share." He was finding it harder and harder to save enough money to reinvest into needed upgrades and salaries for his employees.

At each visit, Glen told of the extreme stress he was under having to work under these conditions. When asked what would happen if he stopped doing the deals, he said, "I wouldn't be able to sell a dowel anywhere in New England." The only enjoyment he got in life was from sports. He played some football in college and was now doing some refereeing for the high school games.

Glen finally sold his business to a bigger competitor. He talked it over with his wife and went for some training and became a professional ref for college football. Between their combined salaries, he thought they would make out OK.

At about the same time Glen's father was starting to have more and more problems with dementia. It was a difficult thing to watch. On each visit, after his mother died, Glen would ask me when he would have to put his father in a nursing home. He couldn't watch him 24 hours a day. "You'll know," I told him, hoping all the time that day would never come. One day Glen came in, and told me he found his father outside in the back yard, in his pajamas, with his gun, shooting at raccoons, and thinking he was back in the war. I told him, "I think it might be time to get him to a safer place, before the raccoons overtake his position and take him prisoner. Of course he'll probably think you've captured him and put him in a prisoner of war camp." Luckily, Charles went to sleep one night and passed away in his sleep before he had to become a POW.

We all have something that we would like to do or to happen before we die. For some it's something grand, like climbing Mt. Everest. For others it's going on a vacation to some place they've never been. Or it may be going back to a familiar place that has good memories. For some it is simpler. It's having the time to say "I'm sorry," or "I forgive you," or "I love you."

Mrs. Beauchemin was such a lady. She was an 80 year old French-Canadian lady, who I had admitted to the hospital. She was dying from lung cancer, and was the mother of a physician colleague of mine at the hospital. He was a pulmonary specialist, with whom I got along quite well. We both had similar political views, and while he loved hockey, in which I had no interest, I would always ask him how his favorite team was doing. When we ate together at the staff dinners, after asking that question, I would then sit back and listen to a play by play description of the last 3 games his team played.

His mom knew her time was short, and I asked her what she would like to do or have happen before she died.

She said something that was quite surprising. She said she would like to have her only child, her son, pray with her. I inquired if she had told him of this request. She said no. When I asked why, she said that she was afraid that if she did, he would never talk to her again.

It seemed her son had fallen away from his mother's faith, had been married outside the church by a justice of the peace and had never returned. He was, in his own words, a devout agnostic, who was not interested in religion or his mother's faith. She was fearful of his losing his immortal soul and, because of this her death would not be peaceful. Then I asked her, if she would mind, if I told her son of her last request, and she said no.

I called her son, and told him I had asked his mother what she would like as her last request before she died, and said I was surprised by her answer. “Do you have any idea what she said?” I asked. He immediately guessed that it was probably that he come back to the church or go to church.

I asked if that was a problem for him. His response was a very strong statement that he did not believe what his mother believed. He also made it clear that the conversation was over.

She died 5 days later with her son at her bedside that whole day. He never said, and I never got the chance to ask him, if he granted his mother her last wish.

A few months later, her son had complications from having a colonoscopy, and died at another hospital. I never got to ask him what he would have wanted to do or have happen before he died, and wondered what he would have said.

In asking this question to dying patients, I found many wanted to heal a relationship or spend time with someone they loved. As one gets closer to death, things become less important, and people become more important. It’s too bad most folks have to wait till they’re dying to discover this.

All the King’s Horses

A chronic nightly problem I had was getting a call from Anne. Anne was a young woman with an old problem—she was an alcoholic. She was a very pleasant woman, and was just wonderful during the daylight hours, but could not control her drinking at night. There was a spell when every night between 2 and 3 AM, she would call crying, telling me what a mess her life was, and I certainly had to agree with her. She was inevitably at a bar when the calls came, and I could hear the clinking of glasses and laughter in the background. She was one of those women who was just unlucky in love. Every time she found herself in a relationship with some guy, it would always end with her being abused, beaten, cheated on and made to feel as if she were of no more value than a whore.

Part of her problem was that she always chose men who would be just these kinds of guys. They even had track records. But Anne was desperate for love and for a family, so she would put up with this until it ended with her being discarded for the umpteenth time.

The sad part was that she was raised to know better. Her mother and father were very respectable and conservative. Her mother was loving and somewhat over protective. Her father didn't ever drink alcohol, but was somewhat distant, and didn't express his love for Anne in words, although he was a very good provider. She was raised in church, and knew what she was doing was displeasing God, and the guilt would cause her to drink. A psychoanalysis would say she was looking for a father's love in all the wrong places. The problem was that her father was raised in a non-demonstrative family that took love and care for granted. It was just something that didn't have to be spoken. It was understood and expected. So he could not give her what he never got, nor what he didn't have. Anne was broken. Once again proving that the sins of the father are passed down to the next generation, even if in a different form.

This was at a time when we had the office phone in our bedroom, and could answer it directly. There was no answering service screening these kinds of calls. When I would say her name, Maria would groan, roll over and try to get back to sleep, while I had an unreasonable conversation with someone who wouldn't remember it the next morning. But I kept answering the phone anyway. I was always afraid that if I didn't, it might just be the one time when she really did need me to answer it. I liked Anne, but I couldn't heal her brokenness. All the king's horses and all the king's men couldn't put Anne back together again. Anne eventually moved away to another state in the South to try to start a new life. I was skeptical of it succeeding as she was also taking all the problems with her. I didn't hear from her or about her for many years, until one day when her sister brought in Anne's obituary. She died of cancer in her 50's, and she was survived by a husband and son. This gave me some hope that perhaps she was put back together again.

CHAPTER 16

Gertrude

One winter Gertrude came into the office. I had taken care of Gertrude since I had come to town, right after her second marriage. She was a lovely Polish widow, now married to a Jewish man. He, being Jewish in nationality only, didn't mind or interfere with Gertrude's love and devotion to the Polish Catholic church which she attended faithfully on Sundays and a few times during the week.

Her second husband was a kindly man and made an excellent companion for Gertrude in her old age. He was the thinker and the reader, while Gertrude was a planner and a doer. After they got married, they moved into her house because she said she had everything just the way she liked it.

Gertrude ended up losing her 2nd husband as well, and made sure to give him a Jewish funeral. Once again she was a widow. When she came into the office, she would talk about all the physical work that was required around her house. When asked if she thought she was up to it, she flexed the biceps on her arms, and would say "strong like bull."

As she aged she began having heart problems—mild heart attack, slight heart failure. After this, the conversations changed a bit. I wanted to know what, and how much work she was doing around her house. She always said, "Not much. I have good neighbors who help me." But I always thought she said this to placate me.

As winter approached, I would warn her not to shovel the snow, and to get someone else to do it for her, as it would be dangerous for her, given her heart condition. After a particularly heavy snow fall, she came into the office that afternoon. The first thing I asked her was: "You didn't shovel the snow. Did you?"

She responded that she had to shovel the snow. I was bewildered. First, I was surprised she survived it, and second, I was surprised she did the very thing I asked her not to do. So I asked her why she had shoveled the snow, when I had told her not to because of her heart condition.

Her response was classic Gertrude. She said, "I got to thinking... because I have this heart condition, I might need an ambulance. So I had to shovel the snow and clear a path to the door from the street. If I got a heart attack or something which would require medical attention, and had to call the ambulance, and the snow wasn't shoveled, they wouldn't be able to get into the house."

I left the room shaking my head, but thankful my predictions were wrong.

Denis

Denis was a neighbor, a fellow church member of the Lutheran church, grew up in Belgium, and married to a lovely Scottish woman. Denis had a large piece of land and loved to work it. He farmed some, cut wood on some and while out there would take his German shepherd dog, Sooner, with him. Sooner would sometimes hunt while Denis would work. The trouble was Sooner liked to hunt skunks. Denis didn't know if Sooner thought they just smelled good, but after an encounter with a skunk, Sooner wasn't fit to be around man or beast.

When Denis was a lad of 8, the Nazis took over his village. He told me that his whole family was put up before a firing squad, for some infraction Denis never understood. He did know that they were not allowed to have a radio or telephone, but they had a radio they thought was hidden. Just as they were about to be executed, his father, who spoke German, got the Commandant to relent. He may have tried to convince the German officer that they were really Germans living in Belgium. In any case his family survived knowing what death and total destruction looked like.

In another wartime episode, while they were in the kitchen of their house, while his mother was cooking, a hand grenade came rolling in. It was tossed in by some Nazis outside clearing the town of traitors. When his mother saw it she ran toward it, picked it up and threw it out of the house before it exploded. When the Nazis, with guns at the ready, came into the house to see who threw a hand grenade at them, Denis' mother began telling them that only she and her children were in the house. Luckily they let them live.

When the Nazis left town everyone thought the war was over for them. In spite of this, Denis' brother did not survive the war. He died one month short of his 10th birthday after accidentally coming upon an explosive device that was left behind by the Nazis.

So for someone who escaped death a few times, and who lost a close brother at a young age, life meant a lot to Denis.

He was not raised in a church. His father didn't have any interest, but his mother was very devout. She had him baptized as an infant, and had him go to a Catholic school during the war, where he learned religion along with math and grammar. Denis learned English by reading the King James Bible and he fell in love with the beauty of the language. The language enthralled him, along with its story of a man who died for him. After seeing friends and relatives die for what seemed like senseless reasons during the war, the idea of a man who willingly gave up his life for others was something Denis could identify with. He knew of many men who sacrificed themselves to save others. And he could understand the totality of the sacrifice of this man Jesus, and he became a believer.

But what one generation experiences cannot fully influence the next generation. How can one take his son to church, have him instructed for confirmation, and by example show how this belief is of utmost importance, and yet fail to pass down the faith to his children, and subsequently his grandchildren? These are questions I had heard many times before by many fathers and grandfathers. Faith is an intensely private and individualistic experience. One cannot make someone believe by force of will or coercion. It is said that God has no grandchildren. Each person must make the decision to follow and obey and become His child. Faith, unlike sin, is not inherited.

Could You Believe What She Did to Me?

Another patient I saw was Yvonne, a 60 year old lady, who had been treated for breast cancer with lumpectomy and radiation. She arrived at the office a month after her treatment because she was "making herself sick." She related that she was "seriously" dating a guy who was "a bit" younger than herself. (A bit happened to be 25 years.) So, make that a lot younger than herself. She and her boyfriend went out to dinner with her oldest daughter and her granddaughter (this daughter's daughter) and the granddaughter's boyfriend. Following the dinner for reasons unknown to her, this lady's "serious" boyfriend dropped her off at home, and then went to the daughter's house with the granddaughter and the boyfriend for a little "party." They all started doing drugs, and while the granddaughter was in the next room having a very intimate moment with her boyfriend, her daughter was doing the same with her mother's boyfriend.

This is what Yvonne was told after confronting her boyfriend, whom she then promptly threw out of her house. (It amazes me how these sorts of guys never seem to have a house of their own or a self-supporting job. They're always free-loading off of some woman.) All the while her daughter denied anything like that ever happened. And how could her mother accuse her of such a thing? Yvonne had not spoken to, nor visited, either this daughter or granddaughter since. However, she worked at the same place as the daughter, so it made for very difficult working conditions.

Since this incident she had an increasing tremor, loss of appetite, trouble sleeping, feelings of depression and outrage. She said every time she looked at her daughter she "sees red." She had been seeing a psychotherapist, who had her write down all her feelings, as well as anything and everything about her relationship and feelings, concerning all her children. Yvonne noted in her write up that this eldest daughter was the smartest and most intelligent of all her children. She expected much more from her than she actually accomplished with her life. The therapist told her that she will never be able to forgive the daughter because her expectations are too high, and her daughter will never be able to meet them. She should just write her off as a lost cause, have nothing to do with her, and get on with her life. (That will be $100, and we'll see you next week at the same time, thank you.)

Her biggest resentment was that her daughter not only betrayed her by what she did with the boyfriend, but also lied to her. She wanted her daughter to come to her, admit her wrongdoing and ask, no, make that beg, for forgiveness. This, it appeared, was never going to happen if her daughter had any say in the matter.

Meanwhile her daughter wanted Yvonne to ask her for forgiveness for not believing her and taking the word of some guy she didn't even know, over the word of her own daughter. Yvonne, from her perspective, wanted to know why this guy would confess to this betrayal and infidelity if it wasn't true.

When I heard this sad tale, I told her I would give her the solution, but she would not want to hear it, and would not want to do it (which immediately caused her to beg me for this solution). I suggested that for her to get peace, and be healed of this, she had to forgive her daughter for what she did, whether it happened or didn't happen. She also had to ask for forgiveness for not trusting her. "Otherwise you will ruin your health, and never have a good relationship with a daughter, who you claim you love, because you're carrying on like a teenager who's love sick over a guy half her age." She said she could never do that. That would be too demeaning. Her daughter is the young one. She should ask her mother's forgiveness.

I agreed with her. It would be humbling, and her daughter should rightfully ask for her forgiveness as well. But we weren't talking about curing the daughter. I asked her if she ever lied to anyone. She admitted that she had. I asked her if she ever had had sex with someone she wasn't married to, and then lied about it, which at that point was a rhetorical question. To my surprise she answered that question quite forthrightly, and admitted to that as well - but with the qualification that "they were all serious relationships."

I showed her that what she had done to and with others was exactly what her daughter had done—lied, deceived and committed adultery. And when God sees her, He probably sees red, too. "Remember the 'forgive us our sins as we forgive those who sin against us' part of the Lord's Prayer? How are your sins going to be forgiven if you don't forgive? Resentment, anger, rage and hate are cancers of our emotions, which destroy us, not those with whom we are angry. It is we who are destroyed with these. If you don't want to be destroyed, this is the answer."

She said she'd have to think about it.

I then asked if she went to a church and she said, "Yes, I go to the Baptist church."

"Great," I said, "talk to Pastor Gil about this and see what he says."

And thought, "It was great to have a clergyman, to whom you could refer these kinds of problems. It sure makes my job easier."

CHAPTER 17

Things You'd Like to Say and Sometimes Do

At a certain point in the life of a practice, one has seen every kind of behavioral anomaly, bad choices and down-right stupidity to last a lifetime. After a while, I would just get so exasperated with some of the things people would do or say that I just couldn't hold my tongue. Here are some examples of things that may or may not have come out:

"Hello! What did you think would happen if you put gasoline on your poison ivy, and then lit a match for your cigarette?"

"You're 14 and pregnant, and you can't understand why your parents don't like your 24 yr. old boyfriend. I'm no genius but I think I can figure that one out."

"You're telling me you failed 4 subjects after cheating on all your tests? Who was the idiot you copied off of? Couldn't you find somebody smart to cheat off?"

"God told you to leave your wife and kids, go to Nashville and start a rock band? You're 50 years old. Has God ever talked to you before? By the way, while He's telling you to take all your money and start a rock band, what is He telling your wife? I hope it's clean out the bank account before your husband gets his hands on it."

"The sign on the fence said 'beware of the vicious dog.' Why did you think it was a smart move to pet this dog?"

"You're 70 years old and have dizzy spells. What in God's name convinced you to get up on the roof? And no, not every bone in your body is broken. Only the important ones."

"Your wife threw you out of the house because you lost your life savings on your business trip, while you were entertaining a showgirl around Las Vegas. And you think that was an unreasonable response? I guess it was. Any reasonable wife would have shot you dead, and collected the insurance money."

"So you went to Mexico, visited the red light district and contracted an STD. Now you want me to fill out a form for you to get a handicap permit for your car? I don't think that qualifies, no matter how handicapped you think you are."

"You're going to take next week off to go on vacation, and you want a note telling your boss that you're sick so it won't count as vacation time. You do realize that I am your boss. I think I'll know."

There was a middle aged guy, who came into the office for a visit, and before he leaves he tells my partner about the new car he just bought. He even had my partner go outside so he could show him around his brand new, just purchased $75,000 car. My partner was impressed, after all he himself drove around in a 15 yr. old dilapidated Chevy Blazer that lost nuts and bolts on rough roads. After this show, he comes back into the office, and tells the receptionist that he can't afford to pay his accumulated $200 bill that's past due. He doesn't have any money, and is just about scratching out enough money to put food on the table and pay off his car.

"But you just bought a new car. Couldn't you see fit to pay your bill that is 6 months overdue?"

"Oh, I've got a loan on the car. I've got to pay that off every month or they'll repossess it. I can't afford doctor's bills."

"What if we called your bill a $200 loan? Would you pay it if we threatened to repossess your kidneys?"

The Philosopher

As one gets older, one experiences the various trials, tribulations and sometimes comical situations life puts you in. There are a number of ways you can deal with them. You can try to control them, which was my first reaction. But you soon find that you cannot control them. They really control you. You can find the humor and laugh at them and at yourself. Or you can become philosophical about them.

When you get married and have children, you think, “I can handle this. After all how hard could it be?” But you don’t handle it as well as you think, so you become somewhat philosophical, and begin to doubt everything you thought you knew. You know you are philosophizing when you hear yourself saying “At least...” a lot. This generally begins as your doctor starts telling you, ‘You’re not as young as you used to be,’ and your kids start their teen years.

My oldest son went through that rite of passage every young man in the country goes through. He bagged his first deer. He got himself an 8 point buck. It was a beauty. Unfortunately, he bagged it with the front end of our car. My son survived but the deer didn’t, and the car couldn’t be saved. “Well, *at least* he didn’t get hurt.”

When my daughter was getting set to go to college, we would encourage her to pick one that would promote high moral values, where there would be good and upright students with whom she could develop lasting friendships; one that would have a good course of study that would prepare her well for a career; and one that would not be too far from home so that she could come home for holidays and some weekends. Where she decided to go was to a school that was 800 miles from home, known for its parties and little supervision. My psychotherapist friend said he couldn’t help me with this. “But, *at least* my treatments would be covered by insurance.”

On her first trip back home from college, at her Christmas break, my daughter wanted to bring a friend to spend Christmas with us. Great, I thought, we'd get to meet one of her friends. Unfortunately this friend was a male, not the female we were expecting. We were to meet this person, an upperclassman, at a McDonald's. As we sat there waiting, we would examine each guy who walked through the door, to ascertain if this was the one. We'd see a number of clean cut, preppy, college looking guys, but no that wasn't the "one." Then a guy walks through the door, who looks like a homeless panhandler, carrying a carpet bag, wearing a very worn and dirty wool overcoat that was thread bear with holes in it. He had long, shoulder length, unkempt hair with a scraggly beard to match. Yup, that was the guy. I'm certain that she chose this guy just to see my reaction, and the look on my face, when he showed up. And I must admit, I must have given her a lot of amusement. "Well, *at least*, she's not marrying this guy."

When my second son decided to take a summer job in New York City, I didn't think it was a good idea. I thought at the minimum he would get mugged, or at least, get his car stolen. Luckily, he didn't get mugged, but unluckily, he didn't get his car stolen—not even with a sign on it that said, "I'm from out of town. Please steal me." So he ended up having to drive it back to college, and continue putting a quart of oil into it every 100 miles. "Well, *at least* it's transportation."

Another son had an intense interest in cars. He studied them. If only he had studied his school work $1/10^{th}$ as much as he studied cars, he would have gotten a 4 year scholarship to MIT. After all this research on which was the best car for reliability, safety, good gas mileage, and was economical to drive, he bought the car of his dreams from a little old lady, who only took the car out on Sunday to go to church. He did pretty well with that car, right up until the right back fender fell off. Seems there was a little problem with the car they didn't tell him about. "Well, *at least* it didn't happen while he was driving."

A very interesting experience occurred while we were visiting colleges. While sitting in our motel room, the fire alarm goes off. As I walked in the hall to see if we needed to evacuate, who should come bounding up the stairs with a fugitive look on his face—my son. "What did you do?" I asked. It turns out he was popping popcorn in the microwave in the lobby, and it suddenly caught on fire and filled the place with smoke. As I got down to the lobby, I saw all these firemen with their combat gear on looking for the source of the fire, and the culprit. While this mayhem was going on, some guy, with suitcases in hand, walks into the lobby, and wants to check into the motel. Now why someone would be wanting to check into a motel that's filled with smoke and firemen was beyond me. Then this guy says, "Gee, smells like somebody burned popcorn. That happened the last time I stayed here." *At least* it wasn't a real fire.

College is also a learning experience for kids. It teaches them how to live with roommates, who when they take off their socks, prompts the entire dorm to go looking to see if something died in the walls, who play bongos at 2 AM, and who have illegal conjugal visits. When my kids went off to college, I discovered that college time is different from whatever time zone you live in. When a 2 or 3 AM phone call starts with, "Hi, Dad, I was just calling to say hello. I didn't wake you up, did I?" "Who me? Of course not. Who in their right mind would be sleeping at this time? What time is it anyway?" You find yourself saying, "What time is it over there because I'm sure it's not the same time it is here." *At least*, they called.

Being a Grandfather

As my children grew up, got married and began having children, I would spend time talking to my patients, who had grandchildren, about the experience. I was told the first thing one has to do when becoming a grandparent is to come up with a name for yourself. And you have to make it easy to say because sometimes the grandchild will change it on you if they can't enunciate it. Grampa can become Grumpy, Grunty, Crampy or just plain Ga.

I found some grandfathers have a great deal of trouble being called Grandpa. They make up all kinds of names so as not to be "labelled" as an old codger. Some names that were used were Skipper, Spike, Big D, The Papster, Big Poppi, Pop-Pop, Big Jake, The big Bear, Peppy, or whatever strikes one as young and hip. I wanted to hold out for Big Jake but I settled for Papa, like the bear.

I also found that when your children have children, you become vindicated. Your kids get to see what you had to put up with while raising them. Plus you get an extra added benefit. You're no longer an old, dull, behind the times dad, who doesn't know anything. You are suddenly transformed into a fun loving, wise, kindly grandfather. You transition from a moron to the genius your grandchildren think you are. You get to hear your kids say: "He let you do what? He would ***never*** let me do that when I was growing up. What happened to the man that raised me? Did he suddenly lose his senses?"

Being a grandfather brings back all those memories of what kids can be like. They can terrorize the cat, eat out of the dog's dish, spill the milk all over the rug, make a box of Cheerios explode, and cover the kitchen and dog in white flour all at the same time. It's just remarkable. It's sort of like watching a physics experiment. No energy is created, it just changes from one form to another, or moves from one person to another, usually going from the parent or grandparent, as the case may be, to the child.

Being a grandparent also makes one a connoisseur of cartoons, Legos, water gun fights, flash-lights in the dark, chocolate chip cookies, ice cream cones and reading books aloud (and making all the appropriate duck, chicken, cow, cat, dog and other animal and non-animal sounds. By the time they're one, you really have got the sounds of ships, trains and planes down pat. And you can do a cow sound so well, that when you do, the bulls come running to you.)

I also found out that you have to tread very carefully around some topics and activities with your grandkids, because if their parents don't like what's going on for a prolonged period of time, they won't let you see your grandkids, which is death to the grandparent (or at least to any relationship with their grandkids.) "Be careful," I was told, "They have hostages. If you ever want to see them again, you'll do as they say."

One patient said after his son had his first child, he up and moved to Wichita, Kansas. Now that's the extent some people will go to make sure the grandparents do not spoil the grandchildren. People used to ask him, "Why Wichita?" He told them, "It's easy. It's equidistant from all the great places you'd ever want to visit or be near. 1500 miles in any direction brings you to some place interesting. And the weather was a veritable paradise—tornadoes in the spring, 150 degrees in the summer, dust storms in autumn, and snow and ice storms in the winter.

Then if he wanted to see them, he'd have to pay a ransom.

"Oh, you want to come and see the kids for a week this June? Great. Jill and I were planning on going to Hawaii for a week, and were wondering if you'd come out to watch the kids while we go."

"That would be fine. We'd love to spend time with them."

"Don't know how much time you'll have with them. We'll leave a detailed list of where you have to drive them, when they have to be there, and what time you need to pick them up. Between school, sports, music lessons, horseback riding lessons and the youth group, we barely see them ourselves. But I'm sure you'll have a good time with them. Oh, and make sure they get to bed by 9 PM each night because they have to be up by 5:30 AM."

"But they're only in the first and second grade."

"Yeah, I know, but we like to keep them busy and expose them to different life experiences."

“Do you think you could expose them to their grandparents once in a while?”

And then it starts.

CHAPTER 18

Who's working Christmas?

As time passed, most of the family doctors joined together into loose coverage groups so that nights, weekends and holidays would be covered without any one doctor having to work every night, every weekend and every holiday. While that was the upside of this arrangement, the downside was the doctor had to cover a much greater number of patients, and consequently, when they were on call, they were working, not waiting at home for the phone to ring.

The Christmas holidays were always rotated. There was Thanksgiving, Christmas Eve, Christmas Day, New Year's Eve and New Year's Day that needed to be covered, and in order to be fair, we all rotated through them year after year. This assured that we would get at least some time off to spend with family at those times.

Christmas was a particularly miserable holiday to work, as working interfered with young children opening presents, family dinners and religious services. It was also miserable insofar as how busy it always was. When working Christmas, whoever was on call was almost always guaranteed an admission or two to the psychiatric ward due to depression or suicidal thoughts, and at least one heart attack or heart failure from either shoveling snow or eating and drinking till they were moribund. Then there were the "accidents": putting the Christmas light someplace where it couldn't be retrieved without the use of an endoscope, getting into a fight and punching a brother-in-law, who now needed stitches, trying to electrocute oneself while putting up the Christmas lights. Then there were the illnesses (sore throats, ear aches, flu, cough, bronchitis, etc.) that had to be cured before

Christmas dinner so they could enjoy it. It never stopped. About the only thing we never saw at Christmas was a snake bite.

So when a husband and wife physician team, who were from India, and were Hindu, came to work in town, the docs thought, "Great they won't mind working every Christmas, and we can always be off." You would think so anyway. When asked if they wouldn't mind working Christmas, for which they could choose another holiday of their choice off, everyone was surprised at the response. "Oh, no, we want Christmas off too." "But you're not Christian, why would you want to be off on a Christian holiday?" "Oh, we have many gods. We don't exclude the Christian ones, so we celebrate all the holidays, including Christmas." Who would have known? It goes to show that when it comes to work, everyone's Christian on Christmas.

Holiday Traditions

When November came, the trees lost all their leaves, the weather turned cold, there was always a threat of snow in the air and people's thoughts turned to the holidays. And like all places, there were holiday traditions.

Obviously, for Thanksgiving, it was the Thanksgiving dinner. Turkey and gravy was a must. Aunt Ida's jello mold had to be there. Also present were Grandpa's stuffed mushrooms, Aunt Connie's string beans and onion ring dish and Cousin Cora's sweet potato and marshmallows. In our house, there also had to be lasagna. The names may be different in each house, but the dishes were the same. And of course there had to be apple, pecan and pumpkin pies. All three had to be there or the desert table was incomplete.

Everyone would say how wonderful everything tasted. Uncle Steve would always say, "Scram gravy ain't wavy," when the gravy came out. When everyone was stuffed and the jello mold was brought out, Uncle Mike would say, "There's always room for jello." Uncle Charlie would then say, "Jello again this is Jack Benny." Cousin Ben would always say how "sweet potatoes and marshmallows make a dinner a feast." All of which they heard either growing up or from some commercial from the 1930's or '40's, but each of those sayings had to be said for the Thanksgiving traditions to be complete. If, as things happened, Uncle Steve or Uncle Mike were not there, someone else would have to pick up the mantle and say it in their absence. It was required for everyone to feel like the day was complete.

The young kids would go out and play football; the older adults would fall asleep after dinner while watching the football game playing on the T.V.; and the women generally would clean up the dishes, put the left-over food in plastic containers and divvy them up to be taken home. Some would play cards or another game. All in all the expectations were low except to enjoy a meal with family and friends.

After the Thanksgiving meal, the grownups would then turn their attention to Christmas. Now Christmas was laden with expectations, so it had to be planned with the precision of a military operation. Whose house would it be at? What time would dinner be? Would they get together Christmas Eve and Christmas Day, or just once? When would the presents be opened? Did everyone want to see the kids open all the presents, or could the kids open their presents at their own home before they came? Was everyone going to go to the same church service?

Unlike the Thanksgiving traditions, the Christmas traditions were much more variable. Each family makes up its own rules. Then there are the arguments. The Murphys always have the same disagreement each year. Mrs. Murphy wants to put the Christmas tree up right after Thanksgiving, while Mr. Murphy wants to put it up Christmas Eve, when he can get a tree at discounted prices. "And don't forget that if we put it up right after Thanksgiving, the needles will be falling off the tree and will become a fire hazard." Mr. Murphy saying that was the tradition in their home. Mrs. Murphy then would counter, "Why buy a tree at all if you're only going to put it up for only 7-10 days?

If we're going to buy a tree, we might as well be able to enjoy it for a while."

The Whites would disagree about which Christmas service they should go to. Mrs. White always liked the one around midnight on Christmas Eve where one was able to get the full effect of the hymns, the organ, the full choir singing and the lit candles. She just couldn't get enough of it. Mr. White preferred to go to the one with less pomp and ceremony on Christmas Day so he could sleep in a little longer. He felt if you've been to one Christmas Eve service, you've been to them all. He was Low Church all the way.

The Keens would argue about whether Mr. Keen would be going to a Christmas service at all. He was not a big fan of Christmas, God or the little baby Jesus and felt like a hypocrite walking into church every Christmas. His wife said, "All the other hypocrites are going to be there. Why should you miss out?" He particularly didn't like it that people would come up and greet him like some long lost soul, who has finally seen the light, and repented of his sins. If he went at all it was just to satisfy his wife. Mrs. Keen was worried about her kids. They were only 11 and 12 and were already asking why they had to go to church when their dad didn't go. Mrs. Keen did not want her children to grow up to be non-church going heathens, like their father, and was going to do everything in her power to see that that would not happen. In the end it was always a 50-50 chance that Mr. Keen would go.

The Willards always disagreed on the dinner. Mr. Willard wanted ham, Mrs. Willard turkey. "We just had turkey for Thanksgiving, and then had to eat it every day for 2 weeks afterward. I'm sick of turkey. Let's have ham instead" was his argument. "But I like turkey, and we only get to eat it once a year at this time. It was our Christmas tradition when I was a little girl, and I'd like to have the turkey," she would counter. Usually after some pretty wet tears were shed by Mrs. Willard, Mr. Willard relented and got on board with having turkey. But he was not happy with it. So, in later years, they would end up having ham and turkey as their family grew.

Then there was the Bernier's oldest daughter, Liz, who just turned 16 and decided this was the year that she was going to become a vegetarian and couldn't eat a Christmas dinner where an animal had to die to provide it. She'd be happy with macaroni and cheese or beans and rice. One thing about a vegetarian is they just cannot be quiet about it. They have to be evangelistic about it, and try to convert everyone else to their faith. She just could not eat her macaroni and cheese or rice and beans quietly and allow others some peace and quiet to enjoy their dinner. So of course, first, she had to make a big announcement at the family dinner table that she had become a vegetarian and that animals have the same rights as humans. Then she had to make a speech, the gist of which was that only cruel, unfeeling, cannibals ate animals, which totally mortified her parents. It was really just political grandstanding, until she started to describe the dirty cages, the blood flowing out of the animal they were eating, while it writhed in agony. That got her father, Gary, started. He said, "I don't think we're killing enough animals. I think we should have ham, turkey, roast beef and venison on the table. The animals certainly don't refrain from eating each other. Why should we?" Liz's 7 year old sister, trying to make peace suggested, "Why don't we just get our food at the grocery store where no animals are killed?" Now it was Liz who was mortified, and their dinner guests sat frozen, looking at each other in stunned silence, wondering whether they dare ask someone to pass the ham.

It's these kinds of interactions that make the ER busy on Christmas Eve and Christmas Day. What is it about Christmas that makes it so stressful? Is it attempting to keep the traditions, or is it the feeling that they are being broken? In any case, the physician on call for the holidays gets to hear about it all.

CHAPTER 19

Iceberg Ahead

I gradually discovered the rules of life:

Rule #1: life will always surprise you with the unexpected.

Rule #2: you will not always like the surprises.

Rule #3: you can't do anything about rule #1 and rule #2.

It was during this time my partners and I were desperately trying to keep our medical practice solvent. All our income was fixed by third party payers, because our payments were either frozen or decreasing. The staff salaries were increasing (unlike, ours which were decreasing), insurance compensation was decreasing, malpractice costs were high, health insurance costs for us and our employees were skyrocketing, and the costs of supplies and services we needed were increasing. It seemed like whatever we did was like straightening the deck chairs on the Titanic. The ship was going down and we were just waiting to abandon ship, and we didn't have enough life boats.

There was the great push on to make physicians convert to electronic medical records, only now the gloves were off, and the clock was ticking. When the idea of electronic medical records was first presented to the doctors, they said if we converted to them, we would be reimbursed more money to make up for the loss of income. That was then. Now it was, if you do not convert to electronic records, you will be paid less than you were getting, and the amount would decrease each year, and we were given 5 years to comply or die.

In looking into this, I found that the cost to implement these records would be approximately $10,000/user, which for us was 9 users—3 doctors, 1 nurse practitioner, 3 nurses and 2 receptionists. Plus there was a yearly "maintenance fee" of $5000/provider. I realized that given our current income, no bank would even give us a loan for the amount of money we needed, because we'd never be able to pay it back. So our options were to opt out of insurance and government payments altogether, or join some other group.

We first looked into joining a large consortium of primary care physicians. This group would be overseen by a board, which would negotiate "the best possible" reimbursements from the insurance carriers. But their best was no guarantee that it would be adequate to keep the doors open. They would also pay for us to hook into their medical record system, but to get this deal, we would have to provide "extra" benefits. The patients' records would be open to them to mine data, and we would be locked into using their labs. For this we would be required to pay an administrative fee of 15%-18% of our gross income. It was a deal they thought we couldn't refuse.

The second option was to become employees of the local hospital, have them take over, and manage the practice, get their medical record system and become salaried employees. The choice was not an easy one to those of us used to being captains of our own ship. We were all used to treating our patients with time, care and consideration. We didn't want them to feel like they were in a mill. We also treated our employees with loyalty and fairness. The employees were all concerned, and with good reason, that they would be replaced, and lose their jobs if the practice was turned over to the hospital. They were all with us many years and their salaries were at the very top of the hospital pay scale.

The third option was to opt out of the third party reimbursement racket altogether. To do so we'd have to collect from the patients directly, who didn't want to pay because they were already "paying for insurance" so "why should they have to pay the doctors?" They didn't understand the desire to cut out the "middle man," and deal directly with us. Some physicians were opening up, what came to be called, concierge or boutique practices, where patients would pay a monthly fee to have unlimited, and anytime, access to medical care from their physician. Some of these physicians would then help file the insurance paperwork for their patients, but since the physician was "out of network," they would not receive any payments from the insurance company. After discussing this model with our patients, it seemed clear our patients were very insurance dependent, and couldn't entertain this financial arrangement.

The time was coming when each physician would have to "choose their own adventure."

If the foundations crumble, what hope is there for the house?

It didn't take a fortune teller to see the decline of our practice, as we had known it. It became quite obvious when my nurse, who had been with me from the start, and my wife, who was our office manager, both retired. My nurse took care of managing the medical side of the practice, and my wife managed the financial side. It was a devastating blow. We were forced to hire a practice manager. It was no longer a Mom and Pop business, and this caused no small upheaval amongst the staff.

It was my wife's encouragement and support of what I was doing that was always critical for me and for any success I had achieved. Without her alongside me, I felt like a horse plowing with a double harness, and the other side empty. It made plowing much more difficult, and it reduced my enthusiasm for the work considerably. Without her there to temper my reactions to all the idiocy that was becoming medicine, I didn't know if someday they'd be taking me out of the office in a strait jacket.

Hiring a practice manager was a new and difficult experience. We placed an ad for someone with some management experience, because none of us had any. Most people who applied had NO experience, not with managing, and not with medical practices. Although, one applicant said she was sick once, and went to her doctor's office, and saw how they ran the practice. That was what she put down for her experience. At least she was honest. Most just thought it would be a cool job.

We finally got 2 people who had some experience, and who seemed like they would at least get the job started, but they also came with a lot of baggage. But picking between the two was like picking between death by fire or death by water. Should we choose the one with anger issues, who was arrested by the police for going after her husband with a meat cleaver? Or should we choose the guy who was fired from his last job after losing their practice a million dollars? And the biggest problem was there was no third choice. I thought I might have chosen Satan, if he had applied. At least he knew how to run a successful business. His operation was still going strong after thousands of years, and was getting more converts and exerting more influence than ever.

We chose the guy. We figured at least we didn't have to worry about him coming into the office one day with a bomb vest, and an AK 47. And he only lost us $500, 000, so we guessed he learned from his last place of employment.

At the same time, the mandates started coming down from the government. Get an electronic medical record system that we can plug into, ***or else*** lose payment. I don't react very well to ultimatums and "or else" statements. At one time it was the physicians who monitored each other for quality care. Then it was the insurance companies (although they were more interested in "cost effective" care, i.e., they don't want to pay for anything). Now with a new president with a new health care bill, the government was going to monitor for what the government cared about. They already monitored our practice hiring for diversity, disability, discrimination and occupational safety. They already monitored for cost effectiveness. Now they wanted information about our patients. They wanted to know who had guns in the house, who smoked, who was overweight, who wasn't using energy efficient light bulbs, who didn't wear seat belts when driving, who suffered from depression, and who was using drugs or alcohol amongst other things. They wanted to be sure everyone had a living will and advanced directives. They wanted to be able to monitor the physician's treatment for "appropriateness of care." In other words, they wanted to make sure the doctors weren't "wasting precious resources" on the terminally ill, now labeled "hopeless," or the very elderly patients (defined as those who were on Medicare). At this point, I felt that retirement was my best option. I could no longer practice in that kind of environment, in all good conscience.

The work environment had really changed. Having an electronic medical record system went from being voluntary to mandatory, and the incentives became draconian. It was like taking the mark of the beast, and everyone knows what happens to those people. And I didn't think I'd do well in the lake of eternal fire trying out asbestos water skis. I liked my environmental temperatures more moderate overall.

Chapter 20

Quo Vadis

With the radically changing climate of medical practice, I began seriously contemplating retirement. But with that came the question: Where would I live and what would I do? I was always told that you have to retire to something and not from something. What could I retire to?

After living in a cold climate, and having to deal with snow and ice (and usually at the most inconvenient times—like when having to drive somewhere), the thought of moving to a snow free or snow less (much less) zone appealed to me. Since we were going through winters with 2-3 foot snowfalls, with the need to have the roofs shoveled to avoid collapse, and $2000 snow plowing bills each time it snowed, I was not viewing cold and snow as my friends. I did not ski, ice skate or own a snowmobile. Winter outdoor activities had no appeal to me. In my younger days I knew older people who tried skiing, and ended up with a broken arm. Or they tried ice skating, and got a broken ankle. At this point in life I wanted to keep all my bones as intact as possible.

Now it may be hard for me to think about Christmas without having to shovel out the car, long underwear, hats with ear flaps, snow boots and jumper cables, but I thought I could get used to it given enough time. Yup, 5 minutes should just about do it.

After considering warm places, it came to be evident that who you lived with was way more important than where you lived. So we decided to move to Texas to be near our sons and their families. We chose Texas over Florida because on our visits to Texas, people were friendly, courteous and kind (for the most part), they had 75 MPH interstate speed limits, and there was a church that seemed like home. Almost all the folks our age had moved to the area from the Midwest to be near their family, just like we were doing. There were good people there with strong Midwestern values. They liked being with friends, drinking coffee, studying the Bible, and visiting. They cared for one another, they took their religion and politics seriously, and they like balanced budgets.

Living in Texas seemed to be very easy. But perhaps the biggest change was in the culture. It was not New England. These people are not like the people we grew up with, and had lived with. New England people see a winter blizzard with 2-3 feet of snow as a test of their manhood. The real men are firing up their snow blowers, and shoveling like madmen to clear a path for their car, which they will immediately take out for a drive in the blizzard, to show that a little snow is not going to keep them home. In Texas, if they get any frozen precipitation, they stay home till it warms up and melts. Don't bother to shovel it. Just sit back and relax. It'll melt soon, and don't go any place because everything will be closed.

In New England, people will chop, split and stack wood all year round, then burn wood all winter to heat their house, so they can brag that their oil bill is less than yours. In Texas, people like burning oil. That's one of their main industries. And energy prices are low. They don't compete with their neighbors to see who can get the lowest oil bill, because they heat with much less expensive gas.

In New England, if someone has a gun in their house or has a permit to carry one concealed, everyone panics. They might call the police, and report you as a menace or a threat to society. In Texas, if someone has a gun or a permit, people are more than likely to ask what make and caliber, compare guns with them and ask them where they go to shoot.

In New England, one could travel through 6 states inside of 3 hours. A long drive is considered anything more than a half hour. If you live in RI, and plan on visiting relatives who live 35 minutes away in MA or CT, you're packing a lunch for the trip. In Texas, folks will drive 3 hours just to get good barbeque. The geographic scope of Texas is huge. The distance clear across CT is about the same as driving from Dallas to Fort Worth. From Boston to Washington, D.C., is less distance than Dallas to El Paso.

In New England, a ranch is a type of a house, and a large farm is 100 acres with cute looking cows grazing in the fields. In Texas, a ranch is a home with cattle, long horned steers and farms that go on for miles.

New Englanders keep things to themselves. Their motto is "good fences make good neighbors." They feel, "It's no one's business what I think, or what I'm struggling with, or what I'm doing." New England etiquette is such that if you meet someone you don't know walking down the street, you ignore them. If you meet someone you do know, you may give them a nod of the head as a sign of recognition. Texas etiquette is such that if you meet a stranger, you not only stop to say hello, you have a conversation about what's happening with them and you. You will find out the most intimate details of the lives of people who are checking you out at the store, bagging your groceries, delivering your dish washer or servicing your internet—where they live, what schools they went to, how many kids they've got, what the doctor just told them, etc. A stranger in Texas is just a friend you haven't met yet.

Some of these differences probably come from the difference in the weather, and from the experiences of our forefathers. Cold weather keeps people inside, and gives one a sense of isolation. In New England, people value rugged individualism. They like the idea that you can do it without anyone's help. They are a people descended from people who left everything they knew in their own country, and fought to establish a life for themselves in a new country with a different language. Their motto is "God helps those who help themselves."

In Texas the weather is warmer and gives rise to more mingling. They still have a sense of being in the Alamo. The idea that we are going to live or die together. We are not alone. We are a people who live in community, and we know one another—who you are, where you moved from, why you came and what you can do—and they look out for one another. Their motto is "Come and take it from *us*."

And in anticipation of retirement, I took up golf. I figured that's what old retirees do, and in a warm weather state, you could play golf all year round. So I picked up some used clubs at a yard sale and a book called, *Golf for Old Guys, Or How to play golf without throwing your back out or tearing your rotator cuff.* I also discovered that it didn't take a lot of practice or lessons to play golf poorly. Anyone could do it, even beginners. In fact if one paid a $20 green fee and played 18 holes and shot a 76, it would come out to 26 cents per stroke. But if you shot a 110, you would find it would be only 18 cents per stroke. Thereby you would actually be playing at a less expensive rate.

I also felt that to really reduce the stress that most golfers feel, that a few modifications of the rules should be instituted. First, one should always be able to move the ball for a better shot. Second, one can carry the ball over water instead of hitting it. Third, anything within a foot of the cup can be counted as in. And finally, never keep score, after all who needs that kind of stress. These modifications will improve anyone's game and make it much more enjoyable.

So Texas seemed a perfect match. Plus Texas was Biblical in the scope of weather one could expect. It has scorching heat in the summer, hail in the winter (just like the plagues in Egypt), and deluge type rains and floods of biblical proportions in the spring. One thing about disasters, it brings people together to help each other, and for pot luck suppers. There's no state income tax, the cost of living is less, you can play golf year round, and the Alamo is the state shrine and Davy Crockett its hero. What's not to like? A more perfect place you'll never find.

What to do?

When I retired, in a way, I felt elated. No fighting with Obamacare mandates, insurance denials or the stresses of medical practice. That is until I realized that now we were also covered under Medicare, and the government will one day decide whether we will live or die. As they said in 1932, "Hey, at least we're not at war, and how long can this depression last?" Lest you're a little rusty on your history, the depression lasted an additional 10 years and ended with the onset of World War II, which resulted in the death of millions of people.

People asked me if I miss "it" without really defining what "it" is. As a male, who generally take their identity from what they do, I would guess in a way I do miss it. But one really needs to know what else one is qualified for and what am I retiring to. I thought about getting a new identity. But the more I thought about it, the more I saw my new identity as being retired.

In fact I thought I had finally found what I was best suited for—retirement. Retirement is the crossing over to the Promised Land, the land of milk and honey. Now I can sleep late (if my aching joints or my bladder doesn't wake me up), travel (if we can ever think of some place we'd really like to visit, and that would be worth the hassle), visit family (if they'll put up with us), and do things that I've long put off (you know those 300 books that you bought, but never got around to reading).

I was once told that God doesn't have a retirement plan. I really don't know if that is totally true. Death is pretty much the definitive retirement, if you asked me. But I do know I should retire from some type of work to another type of work. Some people use retirement to climb mountains, go to the mission fields, volunteer at some homeless shelter or soup kitchen or start another business. While that may be all well and good, I think there's something to be said for taking the time to stand back, get away from all the madness and busyness of the working life, and to contemplate what God is offering us in retirement. Maybe retirement is a time to set things right, that weren't so right before. A time to re-establish relationships that have been neglected. A time to be a better mom or dad, grandpa or grandma, husband or wife. A time to share the wisdom you have gained and experiences you have learned from (not that anyone would listen to an old fool like you, but to try anyway). A time to get to know the Lord better, and a time to listen and hear His voice, now that it's quiet. A time for sharing who God is, and how He has blessed you. A time to help a neighbor, friend or someone who is lonely, depressed, despairing or forgotten. A time to maybe write a book.

So as was written, "Where are the snows of yesteryear?" The pleasure and beauty of this world is fleeting, and the snow covers the dead grass, trees and bushes. But the grass, trees and bushes are not really dead. They are only waiting for spring to come alive again to a new life of beauty and grace.

So retirement may be the ultimate winter experience of life. The snow is coming. Death seems just a heartbeat away, and our dead bodies will someday be lying in the ground. But right in the middle of winter, at the darkest time, Christmas comes. God comes to us with His grace, with His mercy, with His forgiveness and with redemption to all generations who believe. When spring comes so will our new life in the eternity. It makes one hopeful, and hope springs eternal in the human heart.

Made in United States
North Haven, CT
05 November 2026

21790379R00098